Coping with
Alzheimer's Disease and
Other Dementing Illnesses

Coping with Aging Series

Series Editors:
John C. Rosenbek, Ph.D.
Chief, Speech Pathology and Audiology Services
William S. Middleton Memorial Hospital
Madison, Wisconsin

Medical Editor:
Molly Carnes, M.D.
Department of Medicine and Institute on Aging
University of Wisconsin
Madison, Wisconsin

Clinical Director
Geriatric Research, Education and Clinical Center
William S. Middleton Memorial Hospital
Madison, Wisconsin

Coping with Alzheimer's Disease and Other Dementing Illnesses

Mary Norton Kindig, M.A.
Social Worker

Molly Carnes, M.D.

SINGULAR PUBLISHING GROUP, INC.
SAN DIEGO, CALIFORNIA

Published by Singular Publishing Group, Inc.
401 West "A" Street, Suite 325
San Diego, California 92101-7904

19 Compton Terrace
London N1 2UN, UK

e-mail: singpub@cerfnet.com
Website: http://www.singpub.com

©1993 by Singular Publishing Group, Inc.

Second Printing 1996

Typeset in 11/14 Times by So Cal Graphics
Printed in the United States of America by BookCrafters

Library of Congress Cataloging-in-Publication Data

Coping with Alzheimer's disease and other dementing illnesses / Mary
    Norton Kindig, Molly Carnes
        p.   cm. — (Coping with aging series)
    Includes index.
    ISBN 1-56593-097-5
    1. Alzheimer's disease—Patients—Care.   2. Alzheimer's
disease—Patients—Services for.   I. Kindig, Mary Norton.
II. Carnes, Molly.   III. Series.
    RC523.2.C87   1993
    618.97'6831—dc20
                                                                93-2669
                                                                CIP

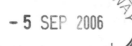

❖ Table of Contents

❖ Dedication

To my father, John Norton, who had Alzheimer's disease and
my mother, Jane Norton, who provided loving care.

Mary Norton Kindig

❖ Foreword

The books in the *Coping with Aging Series* are written for men and women coping with the challenges of aging, and for their families and other caregivers. The authors are all experienced practitioners: doctors, nurses, social workers, psychologists, pharmacists, nutritionists, audiologists, physical and occupational therapists, and speech-language pathologists.

The topics of individual volumes are as varied as are the challenges that aging brings. These include: hearing loss, low vision, depression, sexual dysfunction, immobility, intellectual impairment, language impairment, speech impairment, swallowing impairment, death and dying, bowel and bladder incontinence, stress of caregiving, giving up independence, medications, and stroke. The volumes themselves, however, share common features. Foremost, they are practical, jargon-free, and responsible. Each contains professionally valid information translated into language people who are not health care providers can understand. Each contains useful advice and sections to help readers decide how they are doing and whether they need to do more, do less, or do something different. Each provides evidence that no single person need cope alone.

None of the volumes can substitute for appropriate professional health care. However, when combined with the care, instruction, and counseling that health care providers supply, they make coping with aging easier. America is greying at the same time its treasury is inadequate to meet its population's needs. Thus the *Coping with Aging Series* offers help for people who need and want to help themselves.

This volume, *Coping with Alzheimer's Disease and Other Dementing Illnesses,* is written by two professionals in geriatrics. Mary Norton Kindig has 21 years social work experience helping older adults and their families and is currently a Senior Clinical Social Worker at the University of Wisconsin Hospital's Outpatient Geriatric Clinic. She not only works daily with persons who have dementing illnesses, but she has also had the personal experience of coping with her father's Alzheimer's disease. Molly Carnes, who is also the Medical Editor of the *Coping with Aging Series,* is a geriatrician with 12 years of experience in clinical geriatrics.

If someone in your family has Alzheimer's disease, this book will help you learn about the illness, find assistance, and make future plans. If you are caring for someone with Alzheimer's disease, this book will give practical tips for coping with everyday tasks, safety problems, and changes in personality or behavior. If you need ideas for working together as a family, this book will give you suggestions in words you can understand. No family needs to cope with caring for someone with Alzheimer's disease alone.

John C. Rosenbek, Ph.D.
Series Editor

Molly Carnes, M.D.
Medical Editor

❖ Preface

A dementing illness or dementia is a disease of the brain that affects the ability to think, remember, and perform everyday activities. Alzheimer's disease is the most common type of dementing illness currently affecting more than 4 million Americans.

This book is written for families who are the unsung heroes providing care. It offers practical advice and information to help families as they cope with the many challenges posed by a dementing illness. Although we recognize there are unrelated and hired caregivers, because 70 percent of the care provided to older adults in the community is provided by families, we refer to caregivers throughout the book as family. We also use the term Alz-heimer's disease because it is the most common type of dementing illness and because the challenges of care are similar regardless of the type of dementia.

Because we recognize few families have the time or energy to read an entire book when they are in the midst of the demands of caring for someone with Alzheimer's disease, we designed each chapter to stand alone. Family members are encouraged to read those sections that apply to their current situation.

The book has three main sections. The first five chapters cover the most current medical facts and knowledge available about Alzheimer's disease and other dementing illnesses. The next seven chapters provide practical suggestions for managing and coping with everyday tasks, safety, and emotional issues. Chapter 13 focuses on how the illness affects the entire family. The final six chapters describe organizations and services that can be of assistance.

We suggest that readers select those sections of the book that are relevant to their unique situations. For example, although some families may have few problems with behavior change, for others behavior may be the single most important issue. Keep in mind that just because a wide variety of symptoms are listed here does not mean they all will happen. We also do not expect the practical tips on coping to work in every instance. However, we do hope our suggestions will help families understand dementia and try new approaches to caregiving when needed.

Chapter 1

Overview

Alzheimer's disease has become a household word. It has been called the epidemic of the 21st century, and it is one of the most dreaded illnesses among older adults. The changes in memory, thinking, personality, and behavior gradually interfere with everyday activities and erode independent functioning. One caregiver eloquently described it as "dying by inches."

Incidence of Dementia

The numbers are staggering. According to the Alzheimer's Association, Alzheimer's disease and other dementing illnesses currently afflict more than 4 million persons in the United States. Millions of family members are also affected because families provide approximately 70 percent of the care. For every person with dementia in a nursing home there are two equally disabled persons with dementia living in the community.

Projections are that the number of persons in the United States with Alzheimer's disease will increase to 12–14 million by the year 2040. Alzheimer's disease is the fourth leading cause of death in the United States, claiming 100,000 lives each year. It costs society over $80 billion a year.

Incidence Related to Age

Although dementia is no longer seen as an inevitable part of growing old, the incidence does increase with age.

The Alzheimer's Association reports that approximately 10 percent of persons over age 65 have Alzheimer's disease, however, this figure increases dramatically to 47 percent in the age group over age 85. Because this age group is the most rapidly growing segment of our population, future projections are alarming.

Types of Dementia

As explained earlier, a dementing illness is a disease of the brain that affects the ability to think, remember, and perform everyday activities. Alzheimer's disease, the most common and best known type of dementia accounts for 50 to 90 percent of the dementias. Other forms of dementia include multi-infarct dementia (MID) caused by small strokes (5 to 10 percent) and mixed dementia caused by both Alzheimer's disease and MID (15 percent) (*Principles of Internal Medicine*, 1991).

Impact of Dementia

On the human level, Alzheimer's disease and other dementing illnesses are equally overwhelming. A diagnosis of Alzheimer's disease changes the entire life of the person who is ill. Gradually but relentlessly it erodes the ability to think, feel, work, love, enjoy activities, and care for oneself.

Families, too, are never the same after Alzheimer's disease enters their lives. Think of Alzheimer's disease as a pebble dropped into a pond, with the widening ripples representing the far reaching impact of the disease. It touches everything: relationships, employment, finances, leisure time, and physical and emotional well-being. It requires constant adjustments and poses many challenges throughout its long course.

Although there is no cure or treatment for Alzheimer's disease, the goal for most families is good care that preserves self-respect, assures safety, enhances comfort, and offers enjoyment of life's small pleasures. This book can help families realize these goals by providing information and suggestions to help them as caregivers.

Summary

Alzheimer's disease represents a major health problem in the United States today. Not only does it affect millions of Americans, but each family it touches is never the same. The next chapter provides guidelines for determining when memory loss in older adults is normal and when a medical evaluation is indicated.

References

Alzheimer's Association, 1990.
Principles of Internal Medicine, 1991, Twelfth Edition, Volume 1, Chapter 30. New York: McGraw-Hill.

Chapter 2

Forgetfulness: When to Worry

❖❖❖❖❖❖❖❖❖❖❖❖❖❖❖❖❖❖❖❖❖❖❖❖❖❖❖❖

As both life expectancy and the incidence of dementia increase, fear of Alzheimer's disease becomes a major worry for many older persons. Misplacing keys, forgetting names, or not being able to remember where the car is parked are sometimes interpreted as the beginning of this dread disease. This chapter aims to help families and persons who are forgetful differentiate between normal forgetfulness, which comes with age, and progressive memory change that needs a medical evaluation.

Normal Memory Change

Scientists who study the brain are in agreement that as people age some change in memory is considered normal. Known as "age associated memory impairment" (AAMI), this change is most often experienced as difficulty recalling something quickly, like someone's name or a specific word. Usually the name or word is remembered later. Although AAMI is irritating and frustrating, it is rarely progressive and ordinarily does not seriously interfere with daily life.

Coping with Age-Associated Memory Impairment

Although there is no treatment for AAMI, you can compensate for it by using the following techniques:

- Concentrate on what you are hearing, seeing, or reading.

- Eliminate any distractions or background noises that might interfere with concentration.

- Organize yourself. Find a regular spot to put your keys, glasses, wallet, or purse. Keep a calendar. Carry a notebook. Make lists of things you have to do.

- When you are introduced to someone, repeat the name and/or develop an association that will help you remember it.

- Try to minimize or control stress, anxiety, and fatigue— all of which can contribute to forgetfulness.

There are books on ways to improve memory. Ask at your local library for suggestions.

Possible Causes for Normal Memory Change

Normal memory is also affected by many factors. Often, if any of the following issues are addressed, memory may improve:

- Vision or hearing changes can cause memory problems because memory is dependent on input from the senses. Arrange for an ear and eye exam if you have not had one in the last year.

- Many medical problems can result in memory changes. If you have not had a thorough physical exam in the last year, make an appointment with your doctor.

- Poor nutrition, such as a diet deficient in vitamins or minerals, can contribute to forgetfulness. Inability to chew because of dental problems can be a factor in poor nutrition. Discuss concerns with your doctor, nurse, dietician, or dentist.

- Lack of exercise affects both physical and mental functioning. Many senior centers, fitness centers, and recreation departments offer special exercise programs for older adults. Check with your doctor before beginning any exercise program.

- Social isolation and lack of intellectual stimulation can contribute to memory problems. Most communities have opportunities for continued social or educational involvement through churches, synagogues, senior centers, adult education centers, colleges, or universities.

- Depression can cause memory loss (see Chapter 10 for a complete discussion of the symptoms and treatment). If you think you may be depressed, consult your doctor.

- Excessive use of alcohol or drugs (including prescription and over-the-counter medications) can lead to memory problems. Talk to your physician, pharmacist, social worker, or local drug and alcohol treatment center.

- Stress, fatigue, anxiety, and grief can also affect memory. Short-term counseling and/or support groups may help you through a difficult period.

Abnormal Memory Changes

Memory loss that seriously interferes with daily activities is not normal and requires a complete medical evaluation.

Symptoms of abnormal memory changes include the following:

- Noticeable progression over a period of 6 months or less. For example, instead of forgetting only an occasional appointment, it is now more difficult to keep track of all activities. Forgotten names or events are not remembered later.

- Serious interference with everyday tasks such as managing financial affairs, following well-known recipes, or caring for self. Abnormal memory change may also cause concerns about safety.

In addition to memory problems, other symptoms of early dementia can include:

- Changes in personality or mood. For example, a person who has always been relaxed may become easily frustrated, agitated, or angry.

- Poor judgment. An example would be an unwise investment on the part of someone who has always been astute at financial management.

Although the person with memory loss is sometimes aware of these changes, it is often the family or others in close daily contact who first recognize the problem and take the initiative to arrange for a medical evaluation (described in Chapter 4).

Summary

Progressive memory loss or marked personality and/or behavior changes are not normal parts of growing older and require a medical evaluation by a physician sensitive to age-related changes. The next chapter is devoted to describing how the normal brain works and what goes wrong when a dementia or delirium occurs.

Chapter 3

The Brain

The brain functions like a complex system of wires and circuits, receiving information from the senses and carrying messages from one part of the brain to another. When the brain is not working properly many changes in behavior can happen including memory loss. When this occurs, it is usually caused by a condition called "delirium" or a condition called "dementia" or both.

This chapter discusses the brain, delirium, and dementia. It also reviews the causes of both reversible and irreversible dementia.

The Brain

The brain is composed of over 20 billion nerve cells. Except for some muscle reflexes that are regulated by nerves in the spinal cord, the brain coordinates every activity every minute of the day and night. All of the nerve cells are connected in a complex array of circuits much like electrical wires. Of course, the connections in the brain among the different nerve cells are far more complicated than any electrical wiring system, but the principles are the same. For the brain to work well, each nerve cell and the connections between nerve cells must be working properly. This means that the proper chemical balance must exist within each nerve cell so that it can do its job at the appropriate time and nothing comes between the nerve cells to disrupt their connections.

Anything that disturbs or damages the nerve cells or their connections will interfere with the function of the brain. Factors that interfere with brain function can be mild, such as lack of sleep, or severe, such as major head injuries or large strokes. Some factors are reversible and some are irreversible. Although science has made great advances in understanding the brain, there is still much that remains unknown about the brain and how it works.

When the Brain is Not Working Properly

The symptoms caused by damage to the brain depend on what part of the brain is damaged. Sometimes only a certain part of the brain is not working properly. For example, some strokes mainly injure the part of the brain that controls the ability to move the arms or legs. This results in weakness or paralysis of the muscles of the arm or leg or both and is called "hemiplegia" or "hemiparesis." Some strokes affect the part of the brain that controls the ability to put thoughts into words. When this happens, it is called "aphasia." Some types of blindness result from damage to parts of the brain involved in vision.

Sometimes many parts of the brain are not working properly. When this happens, the brain has difficulty handling the information it is receiving. The eyes may see, the ears may hear, the fingers may touch, but the brain cannot interpret what is being seen, heard, or felt. When the brain is having difficulty handling information properly, it can cause memory problems, difficulty concentrating, confusion, changes in personality, disorientation, and even hallucinations. This can be frightening and may cause agitation as in a bad dream.

When the brain is having difficulty handling the information it is receiving, it is called an "organic mental syndrome." This can be thought of as "brain failure" just as "heart failure" refers to conditions when the heart is not working properly and "kidney failure" refers to conditions when the kidney is not working properly. The most common types of organic mental syndromes are delirium and dementia.

Delirium

"Delirium" refers to a state that comes on quickly (usually over hours or days) in which many parts of the brain are not working properly. Delirium is usually reversible. Anything that interferes in a potentially reversible way with the ability of the nerve cells in the brain to communicate with each other can cause a delirium. It can be thought of as "acute brain failure."

Causes of Delirium

Delirium can be caused by many things. Some medications can cause delirium, particularly when used in large doses or in older persons. Not everyone who takes these medications will experience delirium. But if a person develops delirium, it is important to let the doctor know whether any medications have recently been started or the dosage changed. The following types of medications are known to cause delirium in certain situations:

- Narcotics such as codeine or morphine, which are often taken for pain.

- All sleeping pills, even those purchased without a prescription.

- Alcohol.

- Some blood pressure medications.

- Some ulcer medications.

- Medications taken for depression, anxiety, or any other psychiatric illness.

- Decongestants or antihistamines, including those purchased over-the-counter.

- Medications taken to treat or prevent seizures.

- Arthritis medications containing aspirin or ibuprofen.

Other causes of delirium include the following:

- Any infection (urinary tract infections are the most common).

- Changes in salt and fluid balance such as occurs if someone has watery diarrhea for a day or more, does not drink fluids for a day or more, takes too much diuretic ("water pill"), has kidney problems, or has heart problems.

- A new stroke.

- Too low or too high blood sugar levels.

- Low oxygen in the blood.

- Too low blood pressure.

- A new heart attack.

- Exposure to high levels of certain poisons such as certain insecticides, arsenic, or mercury.

- Liver failure.

Criteria for the Diagnosis of Delirium

The American Psychiatric Association has outlined clinical criteria which, if present, indicate that a person has a delirium. These are published in the *Diagnostic and Statistical Manual of Mental Disorders*, Third Edition, Revised (1987) (DSM-IIIR).

These are the DSM-IIIR criteria for diagnosing delirium and some examples:

A. Reduced ability to maintain attention.

If someone is having difficulty maintaining attention, questions may have to be repeated several times; the person may repeat the answer to the question over and over (perseverating) or answer a question asked earlier in the conversation (intrusion).

B. Disorganized thinking.

This may be indicated by rambling or incoherent speech.

C. At least two of the following:

1. Reduced level of consciousness.

Typically this means a person is excessively sleepy and may have difficulty keeping awake during a conversation.

2. Disturbances in perception.

This means a person is having difficulty interpreting the information coming into the brain from the senses. In mild delirium, a person may be able to report that he or she is not thinking properly or can see things he or she knows are not there. These are called "visual hallucinations." As delirium becomes more severe, the person may be confused, disoriented, and not be able to recognize familiar persons. It may become difficult for the person to distinguish between what is real and what is hallucination.

3. Disturbance of sleep-wake cycle.

A person may be sleepy during the day and unable to sleep at night.

4. Increased or decreased psychomotor activity.

This means a person is either abnormally inactive or abnormally agitated and restless.

5. Disorientation to time, place, or person.

Most often a disoriented person is unable to state the correct date or location.

6. Memory impairment.

D. The features listed in A, B, and C must have developed over a short period of time (usually hours to days) and tend to fluctuate over the course of a day. The symptoms are often worse at night.

E. The difficulties in thinking are caused by a physical (organic) abnormality and could not be entirely caused by another psychiatric problem, such as schizophrenia.

Delirium can range from mild to severe. In severe delirium, a person may be completely unable to communicate. Delirium can be very frightening for both the delirious person and the caregiver.

Delirium Requires Prompt Attention

Because the brain is not working properly in delirium, persons who are delirious are not in control of their actions. This means that harm can come to them while they are delirious. For example, persons who are delirious may fall and hurt themselves or they may choke. To prevent this from happening, relatives should call the doctor at the first sign of delirium, such as a change in behavior or increased agitation.

Delirium is almost always reversible when the cause is removed. Delirium, however, can be a medical emergency, therefore, it is always necessary to call the doctor if you or the person you are caring for develops delirium.

Dementia

Like delirium, "dementia" refers to a state where the brain is not working properly, but unlike delirium, dementia develops more gradually (months to years) and is less likely to be reversible. It can be thought of as "chronic brain failure." In addition, persons with dementia are typically awake and alert, whereas with delirium they are more likely to be unusually sleepy, at least during parts of the day.

It is sometimes difficult to distinguish between dementia and delirium, especially if the person has been delirious for quite some time. In addition, persons with dementia are more susceptible to becoming delirious from any of the factors listed previously. Until a diagnosis is certain, physicians should always look for causes of delirium in a person with confusion or memory problems.

Senility

You may have heard persons talk about "senility" or someone being "senile." These terms were used in the past to refer to an older person who has dementia. It used to be thought that senility was an inevitable part of the aging process. We now know that dementia is an illness that is not part of normal aging.

Symptoms of Dementia

Persons who have dementia have memory problems. They have problems remembering things that have just happened (sometimes called "short-term memory") as well as things that happened in the past (sometimes called "long-term memory.") However, remembering recent events is usually more difficult. The memory problems in dementia are more severe than the problems associated with normal aging as described in Chapter 2.

In addition to memory problems, persons who have dementia may have difficulty with complex tasks that require coordination of several different parts of the brain. These tasks might include driving, dressing, or playing a game. Dementia may affect persons differently but often includes changes in personality, changes in judgment, problems with arithmetic, and difficulty under-standing ideas.

Criteria for the Diagnosis of Dementia

The American Psychiatric Association has outlined clinical criteria that must be present to make the diagnosis of dementia. These are published in the *Diagnostic and Statistical Manual of Mental Disorders*, Third Edition, Revised (1987) (DSM-IIIR).

These are the DSM-IIIR criteria for diagnosing dementia and some examples:

A. Impairment in short-term and long-term memory.

Short-term memory relates to the ability to learn new information. Someone with impairment in short-term memory may be unable to remember the names of three objects 3 minutes after learning them.

Long-term memory includes such things as birthplace, former occupation, names of children or parents, or name of current president.

B. At least one of the following:

1. Impairment of abstract thinking.

   Examples of abstract thinking include recognizing similarities between objects such as "pear" and "plum," differences between similar words such as "right" and "write," or definitions of concepts such as "liberty."

2. Impaired judgment.

   Giving all your savings to someone selling oil wells in Delaware is an example of poor judgment.

3. Impairment in other areas of brain function.

   This includes difficulty using language (aphasia), performing purposeful movements such as dressing or walking (apraxia), and naming familiar objects such as a pen or watch (agnosia).

4. Change in personality.

   For example, a gentle, loving person may become angry and hostile.

C. The problems in A and B must be severe enough to interfere with work, social activities, or relationships with other persons.

D. The person cannot have delirium at the time of the diagnosis of dementia.

E. The difficulties in thinking are caused by a physical (organic) abnormality and could not be entirely caused by another psychiatric problem, such as schizophrenia.

Causes of Dementia

Dementia can be caused by any process that destroys the nerve cells of the brain. The two most common causes of dementia are Alzheimer's disease and dementia caused by strokes called "multi-infarct dementia." The incidence of each type is described in Chapter 1. Some persons have both Alzheimer's disease and multi-infarct dementia.

Treatable Causes of Dementia

Certain medical conditions can cause dementia. Many of these are treatable. Some of the causes of potentially reversible dementia are the same as the causes of delirium. Potentially reversible causes of dementia include the following:

- Side effects of medications listed previously, particularly sleeping pills or pills taken for anxiety.

- Major depression (see Chapter 10 for symptoms of depression).

- A low level of thyroid hormone (this is called "hypothyroidism").

- A low level of vitamin B-12.

- Severe nutritional deficiencies.

- Infections that involve the brain such as syphilis.

- The consumption of large amounts of alcohol over many months or years.

- Tumors of the brain.

- Bleeding around or into the brain.

- Exposure to high levels of certain poisons such as certain insecticides, arsenic, or mercury over a long time.

The evaluation described in Chapter 4 includes tests for these.

Reversible and Irreversible Dementias

The separation of dementias into reversible and irreversible is difficult. Some persons who have irreversible dementias such as Alzheimer's disease may show some improvement when other medical problems such as depression or hypothyroidism are treated. Multi-infarct dementia is no longer classified as an irreversible dementia since research has shown brain function may improve if the risk factors for strokes are treated. Anyone on a blood thinner to prevent further strokes must be monitored closely by a doctor.

Dementias that are generally classified as irreversible are those that are caused by diseases where the nerve cells die at rapid rates for unknown reasons. These are also called "primary degenerative dementias." In addition to Alzheimer's disease, which will be discussed in more detail in Chapter 5, there are some other primary degenerative dementias that destroy nerve cells and cause dementia. These are less common than Alzheimer's disease and differ from Alzheimer's disease in their course, age of onset, and microscopic findings in nerve cells of the brain. These diseases include:

- Parkinson's disease-related dementia.

- Pick's disease.

- Huntington's disease.

- Jacob-Creutzfeldt disease.

Because Alzheimer's disease is by far the most common cause of dementia, the chapters in this book will refer to "the person with Alzheimer's disease." The information provided in this book, however, applies to persons with any type of dementia.

Summary

We now turn from a description of how the brain works to the next chapter for a discussion of what a medical evaluation for possible dementia should include.

References

American Psychiatric Association. (1987). *Diagnostic and Statistical Manual of Mental Disorders* (Third Edition-Revised).

Chapter 4

The Medical Evaluation

This chapter is devoted to the medical evaluation of memory loss and other symptoms of a dementing illness. It describes the reasons for an evaluation, who should perform it, what a complete evaluation should include, and how the explanation of the diagnosis to both the person with dementia and the family should be managed. This chapter is written both for persons who may be concerned about their own memory problems and families who may be the first to recognize early symptoms of a dementia.

Why an Evaluation is Important

If the symptoms of memory loss and other changes described in Chapter 2 are progressive and begin to interfere with daily functioning, a complete medical evaluation should be arranged as soon as possible.

As discussed in Chapter 3, there are several reasons for obtaining an early evaluation:

1. There may be a treatable reason for these changes, such as a drug reaction, low thyroid condition, or depression. The sooner the reason is found and treatment begun, the sooner the person will feel better.

2. Knowing something is wrong but not knowing the reason causes anxiety for both the person with memory problems and the family. Even if the diagnosis is Alzheimer's disease, it is usually better to find out and begin to adapt than to continue to worry.

3. If the changes are caused by an illness such as Alzheimer's disease, everyone in the family will need information. If the

cause is not identified, families will have nowhere to turn for help or advice.

4. An accurate and early diagnosis is necessary in order to make future plans. When an early diagnosis of Alzheimer's disease is made, it is possible to involve the person with dementia in necessary financial, legal, and health care planning.

5. Prior to learning the diagnosis, families often blame the person for the changes they see in functioning or personality. Knowing that these changes are caused by a disease helps families develop more realistic expectations and reduces the anger and frustration they are experiencing.

Resistance to an Evaluation

Frequently, families are the first to identify change in memory, behavior, or personality. It is often difficult for families to persuade persons with memory loss to agree to medical evaluations for problems they do not even recognize. Even if they admit there are some changes, they may blame external events such as a move, job change, or stress in the family. They may state that nothing can be done because memory loss is an inevitable part of growing old. They may resist an evaluation because they are fearful of the outcome. Other people in the family may share these views. All of these factors can delay an evaluation.

Strategies for Resistance

The most compelling argument to use when either the person with memory loss or other family members are resisting an evaluation is that it is important to discover whether there is a treatable reason for these changes. It is also often less threatening to focus on physical changes than memory loss as a reason for getting an evaluation. For example, if fatigue is a complaint, point out that it could be caused by low thyroid, anemia, or a vitamin deficiency.

Another possible strategy is to enlist the help of the family doctor, other health professionals, or people outside the family whom your relative trusts, to support the need for an evaluation. Or you can simply say that you need an evaluation for your own peace of mind.

Who Should Do the Evaluation?

There are many different types of physicians in a variety of settings who can perform a memory evaluation. The most important requirement is that the doctor is interested and knowledgeable about diagnosing and treating persons with these symptoms.

Start with Your Physician

The place to begin is with the doctor who already provides the regular medical care. Discuss concerns, review the elements of a complete evaluation, and determine whether the evaluation can be done by that physician or whether a referral to someone else is needed.

Other Physicians

If there is no family doctor or if the regular doctor refers you elsewhere, these are the types of physicians who most often do memory evaluations:

Family Practitioners: Doctors who see people of all ages.

Internists: Doctors who specialize in the diagnosis and treatment of medical illnesses in adults.

Geriatricians: Doctors who specialize in providing health care to older persons.

Neurologists: Doctors who specialize in illnesses of the nervous system.

Psychiatrists: Doctors who diagnose and treat mental health problems.

How to Find a Physician

The types of doctors just described can be found in private practice clinics, special geriatric clinics, teaching hospitals associated with medical schools, or major medical centers. Sometimes these physicians work with a team of other health professionals including nurses, social workers, or occupational therapists with special training in geriatrics. They may also order special testing from a neuropsychologist.

Call the following organizations for suggestions of experienced physicians or to check references:

- The local Alzheimer's Association.

- The nearest Medical Society.

- The closest medical school or university hospital.

A Second Opinion can Help

If a diagnosis of Alzheimer's disease or another dementia has been made without a complete examination, it is a good idea to obtain a second opinion from one of the types of physicians described previously. It will probably save time if the results of the initial evaluation are brought along. Doctors are accustomed to patients asking for second opinions and usually cooperate by providing the records.

What the Evaluation Includes

As for any medical problem, the evaluation of someone who may have a dementing illness consists of three basic elements: the history of the illness, a physical examination, and laboratory studies. Each is reviewed so that you will know what to expect when you or your family member are evaluated for memory loss.

The History

Taking the history of the memory problem involves collecting information. Usually this is done in an interview with a doctor. The doctor should interview both the individual and a family member or close friend to obtain an accurate picture of the problem. Since memory loss is the hallmark of dementing illnesses, it is usually difficult for persons being evaluated to provide detailed information about their symptoms. In clinics specializing in the evaluation of persons with memory problems, a physician, social worker, and nurse often are involved in collecting information from both the individual and the family. The questions that may be asked of the person with the memory problem and his or her family members relate to the causes of dementia and delirium listed in Chapter 3.

The doctor will be asking questions:

- To determine when the problem began and whether it has progressed slowly or rapidly.

- To look for medical factors such as high blood pressure or head injuries that put the person at risk of developing memory problems.

- To look for dementing illnesses in other family members.

- To look for the presence of depression, which can cause memory problems.

- To find out how severe the problem is.

The history charts the course of the memory problem and identifies possible causes. The information obtained from the history helps guide the rest of the evaluation of the person who may have a dementing illness.

The Physical Examination

The physical examination of the person being evaluated for a dementing illness is almost always performed by a physician in one of the specialties described earlier in this chapter. In some clinics, a nurse practitioner or physician's assistant working with a physician may perform parts of the physical examination. In clinics affiliated with universities or medical schools, physicians in training may perform an examination under the supervision of a senior physician. The examination may vary slightly from person to person depending on information obtained in the history, but it almost always includes evaluation of or performance of the following:

- Weight.

- Blood pressure and pulse while both lying and standing.

- Brief memory test (usually about 30 questions).

- Inspection of ear canals and back of eyes.

- Stethoscope examination of lungs and heart.

- Feeling the abdomen.

- Tapping the reflexes of the arms and legs.

- Testing the ability to feel a pin, a light touch, and a vibration.

- Balance and walking ability.

- Strength.

Depending on the findings from the history and physical examination, some persons may be asked to see a neuro-psychologist for a more detailed examination of memory and thinking ability.

Laboratory Studies

The physician is guided by the history and physical exam-ination in the selection of laboratory tests. However, the following tests are usually ordered in the evaluation of persons with memory problems. These tests were recom-mended by a panel of experts on dementing illnesses at the National Institute of Aging in 1987.

Blood Tests

These are the types of blood tests most commonly ordered.

- Complete blood count (CBC) to look for anemia (red blood cells) and infection (white cells).

- Blood chemistry panel, which evaluates the level of certain salts (sodium, potassium, chloride, calcium), blood sugar (glucose), kidney function, liver function, and often cholesterol in the blood.

- Thyroid function tests (to see if the thyroid gland is making too much or too little thyroid hormone).

- Vitamin B-12 (low levels can cause problems with functioning of the brain).

- Test for syphilis (an infection that can involve the brain).

A blood test for the AIDS virus may be done if the history revealed possible exposure to this virus through contact with infected persons at any time or blood transfusions before 1985. Blood transfusions as of 1985 are virtually free from risk of contracting the AIDS virus.

Researchers are looking for a blood test to diagnose Alzheimer's disease because none is available.

Urine Tests

Urine tests should include all of the following components.

- Dipstick test of the urine for blood, protein, sugar.

- Examination of the urine under the microscope.

- Culture of the urine to check for infection.

Electrocardiogram (EKG) and Chest X-Ray

An EKG is a record of the rhythm of your heart; it may also tell if there has been a previous heart attack. A chest X-ray looks for pneumonia, cancer, or heart failure.

The tests listed above comprise the routine evaluation of all persons with memory problems. The tests described below are also sometimes performed depending on the course of the illness and the results of the physical examination and routine laboratory tests.

For most persons with memory problems who are being evaluated for the first time, the physician will order an imaging study of the brain. There are several types of brain-imaging studies as described below.

Imaging Studies

CAT or CT Scan

This is the simplest of the brain imaging studies. It is a detailed X-ray of the brain. "CAT" or "CT" stand for "computerized axial tomography." The CT scan will show if there have been strokes, bleeding into or around the brain, a brain tumor, or any compression of the brain from a blockage of the flow of fluid around the brain.

These scans are performed by X-ray technicians and interpreted either by a radiologist or neuroradiologist. A radiologist is a physician with special training in performing and interpreting X-rays. A neuroradiologist is a radiologist who has additional training in performing and interpreting imaging studies of the brain.

Sometimes the radiologist will inject a substance into a vein of the person having a CT scan. This substance is called "contrast" because it shows up on the CT scan in sharp contrast to the normal brain tissue. A warm flush is sometimes felt when the contrast is injected. The contrast helps highlight certain parts of the brain so the radiologist can look for abnormalities.

MRI Scan

Sometimes the physician will want to get more information about the structure of the brain than a CT scan can offer. In these cases, an MRI is often ordered. "MRI" stands for "magnetic resonance imaging." It gives a detailed picture of the brain. Like the CT scan, MRI scans are performed by technicians and interpreted by radiologists or neuroradiologists. A contrast material is sometimes injected into a person's vein to further enhance the picture of the brain.

MRI scans are not available in all centers. Sometimes the MRI is helpful, but it is not ordered routinely in evaluations of memory problems.

PET Scans

Other imaging studies are available in some centers but are used mostly for research. For example, PET imaging will show how active different parts of the brain are. "PET" stands for "positron emission tomography." The benefit of PET scanning in the evaluation of memory problems has not been established.

If the person being evaluated has severe memory problems or tends to become easily confused or frightened, performing any imaging study may be difficult. To get a good image of the brain, the person must be able to hold still for several minutes at a time. Both a CT and MRI also require that the individual lie in an enclosed space during the study, which may be frightening for a confused person. If this is a concern for you or the person you are caring for, be sure to discuss with your doctor the specific benefits these tests may offer, and ask how the results of these tests will influence management of the memory problem.

Other Studies

In addition to the tests described, in some instances the physician may want to do other studies. The selection of these tests is guided by the results of the history, physical examination, and initial laboratory studies.

Lumbar Puncture

A lumbar puncture is a test where the physician takes a sample of the fluid that flows around the brain and spinal cord. This fluid is called "cerebrospinal fluid" or "CSF."

Examination of the CSF is especially helpful if an infection around the brain is suspected.

Electroencephalogram (EEG)

An EEG is not a routine part of the investigation for memory problems but may sometimes be useful. An EEG measures the electrical activity of the outer areas of the brain through several electrodes placed on the scalp. EEGs are especially helpful to investigate seizures. They can sometimes be helpful when it is difficult clinically to distinguish dementia from delirium (see Chapter 3).

Neuropsychological Testing

Neuropsychological testing involves a visit with a neuropsychologist. The neuropsychologist will administer a number of standardized tests to see how the brain is working compared to other persons in the same age group. These usually include tests of memory, language, problem solving, vocabulary, and mathematical ability. Neuropsychological testing may be especially helpful when the memory problems are mild or when the cause of the memory problem is not clear and the doctors want to be able to see how the ability of the brain to function changes with time. In this case, repeating the tests in 6 to 12 months might be helpful.

Neuropsychological testing can also help assess the types of activities a person with dementia can still perform adequately. In this way these tests can assist in determining competency and safety risks.

Making a Diagnosis

When all the information from the history, physical examination, and laboratory tests has been collected, the physician will usually be able to tell whether a dementing illness is present, the most likely cause of the dementing illness, and what other medical conditions may be contributing to the problem. It may take several visits to complete the full investigation.

Sometimes, even after a thorough evaluation, the doctor will not be able to say whether a person has a dementing illness. This is most likely in the early stages of a dementia or in persons who are well educated and who may have large vocabularies and memory stores. Because such persons usually function above average, it takes longer for problems with brain function to come apparent. In these instances, neuropsychological testing can be particularly helpful. If after neuropsychological testing the diagnosis of a dementing illness is still in question, repeating these tests in 6 to 12 months will usually confirm whether a person's brain is affected by a progressive dementing process.

Some diseases of the brain can only be diagnosed definitively by looking at a piece of the brain under the microscope. Because taking a piece of the brain from persons while they are alive is rarely done and then only as part of research studies, the definitive diagnosis of diseases such as Alzheimer's disease can only be done after death by an autopsy (see Chapter 19). However, from the history, physical examination, and laboratory studies, the physician will make the correct diagnosis about 80 percent of the time. Reevaluating the course of the memory problem approximately every 6 months can also help the physician make the correct diagnosis.

Explanation of the Diagnosis

The way in which the diagnosis is explained should be planned in advance with the doctor, the person being evaluated, and the family. It should always take place in a face-to-face meeting; learning the diagnosis on the telephone or in a letter does not provide the necessary opportunity for questions, discussion, and support. Make sure there will be enough time to ask questions, share feelings, and discuss recommendations.

What the Explanation Should Include

For everyone to understand how the diagnosis was made, the doctor should review the process of the evaluation and the results. This is especially important if the diagnosis is Alzheimer's disease, because everyone will want to be assured that all other possible explanations have been carefully evaluated and excluded. Whatever the diagnosis, it should be presented in a clear and straightforward manner. Although it is painful and distressing to hear the words "Alzheimer's disease," it is necessary to know the diagnosis to make realistic future plans. Also, without a diagnosis, the family will have difficulty understanding and coping with the inevitable behavior and personality changes that will occur.

Topics for Discussion

Here are some of the issues that should be covered in the meeting:

- What should the person with dementia be encouraged to do independently?

- What supervision is needed?

- What activities, if any, are no longer safe?

- What community services might be helpful?

- Is the person competent to sign important legal documents (see Chapter 14)?

Involving the Person with Dementia

It is usually advisable for the person with a dementing illness to be included in the meeting where the diagnosis is presented for the following reasons:

- People have a right to information about their medical conditions.

- Persons with a dementing illness need to be involved as much as possible in decisions and plans about their lives and future.

- If the person is excluded, talking openly about the illness and its consequences becomes difficult, if not impossible.

Persons with Alzheimer's disease and other dementias may have trouble grasping complicated explanations. However, that in itself is not a reason to exclude them from the discussion. It does necessitate presenting the information clearly and simply and allowing enough time for questions and further explanations.

There may be a few instances in which it is not a good plan to include the person with Alzheimer's disease in the meeting with the doctor. These might include situations such as the following:

- If the diagnosis is tentative and a repeated evaluation in 6 to 12 months is needed to confirm it.

- If the person with dementia is at high risk of depression and/or suicide.

- If the person with dementia is suspicious and would likely interpret the meeting as a plot.

- If the diagnosis is made late in the disease and the person with a dementing illness is too confused to understand even the simplest explanation.

In all cases, however, these exceptions should be discussed in advance with the doctor.

Including the Family

Because this is an illness that will affect everyone in the family, it is important for as many family members as possible to attend the meeting with the doctor so that everyone hears the same information. A telephone conference call can be used to include family members who live at a distance.

There may be times throughout the course of the illness when family members need to speak privately with the physician or with other health care providers. This issue is addressed in Chapter 15.

Reactions to the Diagnosis

Dealing with a devastating diagnosis such as Alzheimer's disease takes time. Everyone may be too upset at first to think clearly. Other questions or concerns will come to mind after the initial meeting is over. If the explanations, diagnostic process, or any of the medical terms are confusing, ask for clarification or a follow-up meeting.

People respond to hearing a diagnosis of a terminal illness such as Alzheimer's disease in their own individual ways. Normal reactions include shock, denial, anger, sadness, anxiety, frustration, guilt, and depression. Each person's initial reaction also evolves and changes with time. For example, denial of bad news often initially keeps people from feeling totally overwhelmed. Eventually, however, denial is usually replaced by anger, grief, and acceptance of something that cannot be changed.

Reaction of the Person with Dementia

The person with Alzheimer's disease or another dementing illness may have more difficulty accepting the diagnosis than other family members. This may not be denial but may be a symptom of the disease that impairs the ability to think, remember, or process new information. If this is the case, arguing or confronting will not be helpful.

Some persons with dementia, especially in the early stages, become severely depressed and even suicidal on learning the diagnosis. This is always a risk when informing someone about a terminal illness. Contact the doctor immediately if there are any indications of depression or suicide. Chapter 10 describes the diagnosis and treatment of depression.

Reaction of the Family

Individuals within the family may react differently to the diagnosis of Alzheimer's disease, causing stress and conflict at a time when everyone needs support. One person may have anticipated the diagnosis while for another the diagnosis is a total surprise. When some people in the family are ready to make specific future plans and others have not yet accepted the diagnosis, it is difficult to move forward. Simply allowing everyone time to adjust often helps. However, if family members continue to hold widely divergent views about the nature of the problem, asking for professional advice from the doctor, nurse, or a social worker may be useful.

Reaction of Friends

It is important to share the diagnosis with friends so they will understand the changes that occur and provide support, assistance, and opportunities for continued involvement and social stimulation. See Chapter 8 for further discussion.

Summary

The main message of this chapter is that a thorough evaluation by an experienced physician is needed to make the diagnosis of dementia. Alzheimer's disease, the most common dementing illness, is described in detail in the next chapter.

Chapter 5

Alzheimer's Disease

This chapter discusses what Alzheimer's disease is and theories for its cause.

What is Alzheimer's Disease?

As described in Chapter 3, Alzheimer's disease is a primary degenerative dementia. This means that many of the nerve cells in the brain stop functioning correctly, degenerate, and die. When enough of these cells die, the brain cannot work properly, and the person develops dementia. At this time there is no test to diagnose Alzheimer's disease. Instead, the diagnosis of Alzheimer's disease is called a "diagnosis of exclusion," meaning that a person has had a complete evaluation for other causes of dementia and none were found. However, when the clinical diagnosis of Alzheimer's disease is compared with brain biopsy or autopsy studies, the clinical diagnosis is correct approximately 80 percent of the time.

The disease was named after Alois Alzheimer who described the first case of this dementing illness in the early 1900s. Dr. Alzheimer recorded the clinical course of the disease in a patient and, after the patient died, he observed the microscopic findings in the brain.

Inherited Form of the Disease

It appears that about 10 percent of persons who get Alzheimer's disease inherit it from their parents. This is called "familial Alzheimer's disease." Persons with familial Alzheimer's may develop the disease at an early age (in their 50s or 60s) and usually have a rapid progression. They may die within 7 years of the diagnosis of the disease. Abnormalities of certain chromosomes have been found in familial Alzheimer's. A chromosome contains DNA which determines the unique genetic make-up of every person. Humans have 46 chromosomes. Some studies have found abnormalities in chromosome 19 and some in chromosome 21. It is interesting that chromosome 21 is the same chromosome that is abnormal in Down syndrome and that persons who have Down syndrome are very likely to develop Alzheimer's disease at an early age. Although genetic testing for chromosomal abnormalities may be performed in special laboratories, this test is not widely available and is not used routinely. However, if you have parents or other close relatives who have developed Alzheimer's disease relatively early in life, you may wish to discuss genetic testing with your doctor. Refer to Chapter 14 for a discussion of possible legal implications of such testing.

Incidence of Alzheimer's Disease Increases with Age

Most persons who get Alzheimer's disease do not have the inherited form. The likelihood of developing the disease increases with age. Although early symptoms of memory problems may begin in the mid to late 70s, in many persons the disease does not begin until the late 80s or even 90s. The course of the disease varies a great deal from one person to another.

Although Alzheimer's disease causes progressive deterioration of brain function as nerve cells die, many older persons who get the disease may remain on a "plateau" for a number of years. That is to say, someone may stay in the early stage for up to 10 years where memory problems are the major symptom. These persons are likely to die of some other medical problem such as heart disease or cancer rather than Alzheimer's disease.

What Causes Alzheimer's Disease?

Alzheimer's disease is "idiopathic," which is a scientific term meaning the cause is unknown. Some of the main theories about the cause of Alzheimer's disease are:

The Virus Theory

According to this theory, the brain becomes infected by a virus or a "prion," which is even smaller than a virus. The virus or prion slowly destroys brain cells.

The Immune Theory

The immune system allows the body to destroy foreign substances that enter it. It enables the body to fight off an infection and heal after an injury. Sometimes in the process of fighting off foreign substances, normal cells are destroyed as well. Some scientists suspect that in Alzheimer's disease, the blood vessels in the brain allow substances from the blood to enter the brain that would ordinarily not be found there. These substances are viewed by the immune system of the brain as foreign substances that must be destroyed. The brain immune system is activated to destroy the invading substances, and normal brain cells are destroyed in the process.

Supporters of this theory point out that persons, such as boxers, who have had head injuries are more likely to get a degenerative dementia, which looks like Alzheimer's disease. The blood vessels of the brain may leak for a time after a head injury, which may even cause bleeding into the brain. According to the immune theory, this would activate the immune system of the brain and result in destruction of normal brain cells in the process.

The Aluminum Theory

Some scientists have found that the brains of persons with Alzheimer's disease contain aluminum. Aluminum and certain other metals can cause damage to nerve cells, but scientists are not sure if this is a cause of Alzheimer's disease or one of its effects. Although there is no evidence that the use of aluminum cooking pots increases the risk of Alzheimer's disease, avoiding exposure to high doses of aluminum is prudent.

The Microtubule Theory

Every nerve cell has a network inside it of tiny tubes called "microtubules." The microtubules are necessary for movement of substances from one part of the cell to another. This movement is crucial for the normal function of nerve cells, which have to carry information rapidly from one part of the brain to another. These microtubules are abnormal in many nerve cells of the brains of persons with Alzheimer's disease.

The Amyloid Theory

"Amyloid" refers to a substance that forms inside cells when something goes haywire with the protein-forming machinery of that cell. Amyloid is made up of many copies of the same protein, which stick together. When amyloid forms in nerve cells, the cells may be unable to function and eventually die. Amyloid has been found in abnormally large amounts in the brains of persons with Alzheimer's disease.

The Acetylcholine Hypothesis

In the late 1970s, researchers discovered that the brains of persons with Alzheimer's disease had a dramatic loss of a certain type of nerve cell. These nerve cells make a chemical called "acetylcholine." Acetylcholine is needed for communication between many of the nerve cells in the brain, especially those nerve cells involved in learning and memory called "neurotransmitters." It is now known that many neurotransmitters, not just acetylcholine, are low in the brains of persons with Alzheimer's disease.

Under the Microscope

Whatever the cause of Alzheimer's disease, it can be diagnosed definitively only by studying thin slices of brain tissue under the microscope. As discussed in Chapter 4, this requires a brain biopsy, which is usually performed only as part of research studies or examination of the brain after a person has died.

To say that a brain was affected by Alzheimer's disease, the pathologist applies special stains to the thin slices of brain tissue and must observe the abnormalities described below in the brain slice. All of these abnormalities can be seen in the normal aging brain as well (see the illustration on p. 52). In fact, they appear to be present in all persons over the age of 90. The difference is that in the brain with Alzheimer's there are more of these abnormalities than in the normal aged brain.

The Neurofibrillary Tangle

Neurofibrillary tangles can be seen with special stains under the microscope within many nerve cells in Alzheimer's disease. These tangles may represent degenerating microtubules. These tangles must be seen by the pathologist to say that a brain was affected by Alzheimer's disease.

The Neuritic Plaque

Neuritic plaques can also be seen with special stains under the microscope in thin slices of brain in Alzheimer's disease and in lesser amounts in normal aged brains. These plaques are made up of a core of amyloid surrounded by pieces of degenerating nerves and certain cells of the brain immune system. The presence of neuritic plaques is also necessary for the pathologist to diagnose Alzheimer's disease definitively.

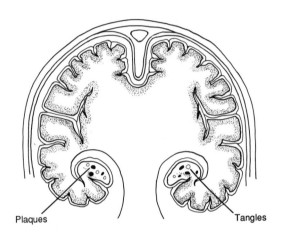

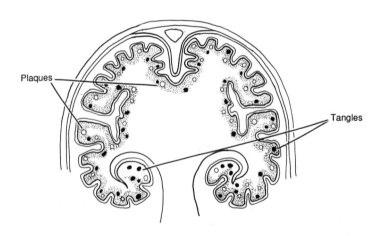

Comparison of a normal brain (top) and a brain affected by Alzheimer's disease (bottom)

Large numbers of neurofibrillary tangles and neuritic plaques are considered the hallmark of Alzheimer's disease (see the illustration on this page).

Research in Alzheimer's Disease

Research is occurring on many aspects of Alzheimer's disease. Methods to improve the ability to diagnosis and manage the disease are being investigated. Currently there is no medication to reliably improve brain function in persons with Alzheimer's disease. Nor is there any medication known to slow the course of the disease. There are, however, many ongoing clinical trials that are

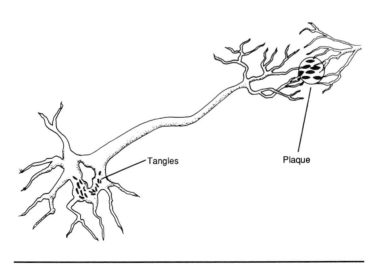

Brain cell degenerating from Alzheimer's disease

investigating a number of different drugs to assess their benefit in treating persons with Alzheimer's disease.

Probably the largest class of drugs being investigated are those that would affect the nerves that use acetylcholine. Because the brain in Alzheimer's disease has lost this chemical, the hope is that replacing this chemical or similar chemicals might help the brain to function better.

Tetrahydroaminoacridine (THA) or tacrine is one of these drugs. It helps increase acetylcholine activity in the brain. However, it has not been shown to reliably benefit persons who have Alzheimer's disease, and many persons get liver damage from this drug.

Persons who have Alzheimer's disease may be asked whether they wish to participate in research projects. Some may involve testing drugs for the treatment of the disease, others may involve blood tests or interviews. Any research involving persons has been reviewed and approved by a committee of individuals established to ensure the rights and safety of research subjects. Additionally, experimental drugs have been approved by the Federal Drug Administration.

The following are factors to consider if you or your family member are asked to participate in a treatment study for persons with Alzheimer's disease:

- A thorough evaluation and close follow-up by experts in the field of Alzheimer's disease is usually included and offered free.

- The medication being tested may turn out to be beneficial, which would help you and your family member as well as others with the disease.

- This is something that may help others with Alzheimer's disease in the future.

Depending on the type of treatment study, the following are reasons some may choose not to participate in a study:

- Extensive testing, especially if it requires admission to a hospital, may be frightening and exhausting for the person with Alzheimer's disease.

- Complying with the demands of the research may add additional burden at a time when you are already feeling overwhelmed.

- The medication under investigation may have unwanted side effects.

Before agreeing to participate in a study, a consent form will be given detailing what is expected in the study and the hazards and potential benefits of the research. In the early stages of dementia, persons with Alzheimer's disease may understand and sign the consent form themselves. In later stages, this decision will be up to the legal guardian (see Chapter 14). In either case, the consent form should be reviewed carefully and any questions or concerns about the research should be discussed with the person responsible for the study. If the study involves a drug, it is a good idea to discuss the study with your family doctor or the doctor who best knows the person with dementia.

If you are interested in finding out about research in your community, contact the nearest Alzheimer's Association, university, or medical school.

Prevention of Alzheimer's Disease

Because the cause of Alzheimer's disease is unknown, there is little that can be done to prevent it. However, Alzheimer's disease is more likely to occur in persons who have had head trauma or injury to the brain. Therefore, everyone should avoid boxing or street fighting and wear seat belts in cars and helmets when bicycling and motorcycling.

As mentioned in Chapter 3, the second most common cause of dementia is stroke, which causes multi-infarct dementia. This type of dementia can be prevented by having blood pressure checked regularly and having it treated if it is elevated. High blood pressure causes strokes. If atrial fibrillation (irregular heart beat) is a problem, ask your doctor about treatment with blood thinners.

Stages of Alzheimer's Disease

Alzheimer's disease is a progressive illness that follows a fairly predictable pattern. Understanding this pattern is important for the following reasons:

- To help develop realistic expectations of what a person with Alzheimer's disease can do at each stage.

- To assist in deciding what community services might be helpful.

- To enable family members to adapt to the challenges posed by each stage.

- To anticipate or reduce future crises by planning ahead.

Alzheimer's disease is often described in terms of three stages. These are not precise categories, and there is a great deal of overlap between them. No two people progress through these stages at exactly the same rate or with identical symptoms.

Early Stage: Forgetfulness

The first symptoms of Alzheimer's disease are very subtle. In fact, early in the illness families and persons with memory problems frequently do not realize anything is wrong. If the symptoms are noticed, they are often incorrectly attributed to old age.

The early stage is called the "Forgetfulness Stage" because a memory problem is often the first symptom. Asking the same question repeatedly, losing things, forgetting appointments or birthdays, or neglecting to pay bills are all common behaviors at this stage. Memory aides such as calendars and lists are often successfully used at first to compensate for these difficulties. However, eventually these techniques cease to be effective.

At this early stage a person with Alzheimer's disease can usually function independently in any environment. Although good days outnumber bad days, tasks that were once easy now take much more effort and learning new information becomes increasingly difficult. Often the individual does not acknowledge problems and may resist help.

Other symptoms of the early stage may include:

- Increased frustration or anxiety.

- Depression.

- Loss of interest in outside activities.

- Difficulty concentrating.

- Problems finding the right word.

- Withdrawal from social situations.

- Blaming others.

- Poor judgment.

Middle Stage: Confusion

As Alzheimer's disease progresses, the person enters the "Confusional Stage." In this stage the person needs supervision to function in familiar surroundings but is usually still able to respond to simple directions. Complex tasks involving a series of steps such as getting dressed or cooking a meal become increasingly difficult. Memory loss is much more pronounced, is no longer helped by reminders, and may lead to such behavior as forgetting to eat. Loss of attention to social conventions such as not dressing properly in public may occur. Confusion about time and place is common. Safety is often a major concern at this stage. Getting lost, leaving the stove on, driving unsafely, and mixing up medications are all common.

Other symptoms of the middle stage may include:

- Neglect of appearance and hygiene.

- Rapid mood changes including fear, anger, or anxiety.

- Depression or apathy.

- Suspicion of others.

- Lack of sensitivity to the needs of others.

- Restlessness, agitation, or wandering.

- Increased difficulty recalling names or words.

- Sleep disturbances.

- Poor judgment.

- Weight loss.

- Loss of bladder control.

- Difficulty swallowing.

This is a difficult stage for families, because the person with Alzheimer's disease is often unable to comprehend what is happening and may resist assistance and/or blame others. Constant supervision is usually needed, which is almost always difficult for either an individual caregiver or an entire family to provide without outside assistance.

Late Stage: Terminal

During the last or "Terminal Stage" of the disease, memory loss and confusion are severe. Sometimes the person with Alzheimer's disease no longer recognizes family. Coordination problems cause difficulty in walking, standing or rising from a chair, and falling becomes a major risk. Loss of bowel and bladder control is common. Frequently the person cannot swallow solids or liquids and becomes malnourished and dehydrated. Eventually the person becomes bedridden and needs total care. Often nursing home placement is necessary.

Other symptoms of this stage may include:

- Restlessness and agitation.

- Hallucinations or delusions.

- Extreme suspicion of others.

- Sleep disturbances.

- Extreme difficulty with communication.

- Compulsive acts such as picking at clothing.

- Withdrawal.

- Seizures.

Summary

Understanding the stages and the progressive nature of Alzheimer's disease is necessary to appreciate how it influences daily tasks and hygiene as well as social and leisure activities, which are the topics of the next three chapters.

Chapter 6

Performing Daily Tasks

This chapter looks at everyday tasks. It provides general guidelines for assessing the ability of a person with Alzheimer's disease to perform daily tasks and offers suggestions to families for encouraging appropriate independence. It describes ways to handle routine activities such as dressing, eating, walking, and household management.

Problems with Daily Activities

A person with a progressive dementing illness will increasingly have problems performing daily tasks. Even a simple routine task, such as setting the table, is composed of a series of steps that need to be performed in a certain order. Persons with dementia have progressively more difficulty remembering and following the sequence as well as learning new behaviors to compensate.

The Diagnosis is Helpful

Because people with an early dementia look healthy and have good social skills, it is easy for others to conclude that they are just "lazy" when they have difficulty with everyday tasks. Establishing a diagnosis should help everyone understand that it is the illness that is causing changes to occur.

Balancing Independence and Dependence

The diagnosis of Alzheimer's disease does not suddenly rob the person of all independence. Families are faced with the challenge of continually assessing the person's ability to perform everyday activities. If expectations are too high, frustration and anxiety will result. If expectations are too low, the person will be denied the opportunity to succeed and may lose the ability to perform a given task, resulting in unnecessary dependence, loss of self-esteem, and more work for the caregiver.

Balancing appropriate assistance and encouraging independence is complicated by day-to-day normal fluctuations in abilities. On "good days" a person with Alzheimer's disease may be even more self-sufficient than usual; on "bad days" the same person will need extra assistance. This lack of predictability is often frustrating for families and calls for both flexibility and patience.

Assessment of Daily Tasks

The ability to perform everyday tasks is affected by physical or medical factors, the person's surroundings, and communication problems as well as the task itself. All need to be taken into account.

Evaluate Each Task Separately

The ability to perform specific activities is often uneven. For example, a person who has always kept a spotless home may continue to be an excellent housekeeper until late in the disease, but in the early stage of the illness the same person may have difficulty dressing. For this reason each task needs to be analyzed separately. Ask whether the person is able to:

- Initiate a task independently?

- Initiate a task in response to cues or demonstrations?

- Finish a task if someone else begins it?

As an illustration of the above, imagine that you are asking your family member for help making a salad. If you ask her to help tear up lettuce, is she able to open the refrigerator, select the lettuce, find the salad bowl, and begin? If not, if you arrange the lettuce and the salad bowl on the counter, will she then be able to begin? Or if you start to tear up the lettuce, will she be able to finish the project?

The Need for an Objective Analysis

It is often hard for caregivers to find the time or energy to analyze each activity. It is also difficult when you are in the midst of a situation to step back and look at it objectively. The experiences of other people in a support group, views of family or close friends, or the advice of experienced professionals such as a social worker, nurse, or occupational therapist may help you gain a different perspective and learn new approaches (refer to Chapter 16).

Planning Daily Activities

When planning daily activities, keep in mind the following suggestions:

- Focus on abilities rather than on limitations as much as possible. Provide honest praise and encouragement.

- A predictable daily routine is important. It decreases anxiety and reduces the need to adapt to change.

- Many self-care tasks are almost automatic and will be retained longer if they are used every day.

- Break down tasks into simple steps. Provide one-step-at-a-time instructions or cues and use short words and simple sentences.

- Accept that each daily task will gradually take more time to do as the disease progresses.

- Encourage activities that have little risk of failure. Give credit for trying rather than for completing a task.

- Reduce distractions such as background noise to improve the ability to concentrate on a task.

- Remember that even simple activities can bring a sense of achievement and/or can promote companionship.

- Allow the person to make choices to improve self-esteem. Confusion, anxiety, or agitation in response to a choice are clues that making that particular decision may be too difficult.

- People with dementia are highly sensitive to the moods of people around them. Try to remain calm and patient and avoid criticism.

- Early fatigue and a short attention span are common in persons with Alzheimer's disease and other dementing illnesses. When possible, plan activities at the best time of day and allow time for rest.

• Rushing a person with dementia often increases confusion, anxiety, or agitation.

Dressing

Causes of dressing problems include short attention span, fatigue, anxiety, and distractions in the home. Subtle changes in dressing, such as selecting inappropriate clothes, often occur in the early stages of dementia. As in most everyday activities, dressing involves a series of steps that include: remembering that it is time to dress, selecting proper clothes, and putting the correct number of items on in the right order (see the illustration on this page). It also requires physical and manual dexterity which is gradually lost as the illness progresses.

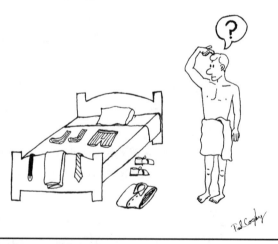

The challenge of dressing

If problems with dressing occur, analyze which step is posing the difficulty and intervene only in that part of the process. A verbal cue may be all that is needed ("maybe that sweater would be warmer"). It may be necessary to begin the sequence such as laying out the clothes in order or, in the later stage of the illness, to help with dressing. The goal in dressing, as in all daily activities, is to maintain as much independence as possible. Maintaining a regular morning and bedtime schedule is helpful.

Coping Strategies for Dressing

Here are some strategies to try if dressing becomes a problem:

1. *Forgetting to dress.* Try laying out the clothes, getting dressed with the person, or giving a reminder ("it's morning now so let's get dressed").

2. *Inability to decide what to wear.* Try decreasing the number of choices by removing out-of-season or infrequently worn clothes from the closet, allowing more time for decisions, or providing verbal cues ("the blue shirt would look nice with those pants").

3. *Insistence on wearing the same clothes every day.* Try buying identical outfits so you can switch and launder them.

4. *Refusal to undress at night.* Try laying out pajamas or a nightgown or drawing the bath water, which may trigger getting undressed. Investigate whether the room temperature is too cold.

5. *Difficulty with the sequence of dressing.* Try reminders ("your shirt goes on next"), laying out clothes in order or,

if necessary, handing the person the individual items one at a time.

6. *Putting on too many items.* Try verbal cues ("you already have your blouse on") or laying out the clothes ahead of time.

7. *Loss of coordination.* Try loose-fitting outfits such as clothes that are one size larger or jogging suits, pull-on pants and skirts, clothes and shoes with velcro fasteners, tube socks, and cardigans instead of pullovers. J. C. Penny and Sears both have special catalogs for clothes of this type.

Eating

There are no special diets or vitamin supplements that will cure someone with Alzheimer's disease. However, poor nutrition can make confusion and disorientation worse and can lead to additional medical problems.

Eating is affected by factors such as cavities, poorly fitting dentures, medications, or constipation causing loss of appetite. The appetite may wane as taste or smell diminish. Seeing food may be difficult with vision problems. Dehydration can result from loss of the sense of thirst. Forgetting to eat or eating all the time are both direct consequences of memory loss. Voicing food likes and dislikes may be difficult when there are communication problems. Using utensils is affected by loss of coordination. Medical problems such as pneumonia can cause loss of appetite.

Try to maintain a predictable relaxed meal schedule and reduce distractions at meal time. Plan a balanced diet and make sure fluid intake is adequate (6 to 8 glasses of any fluid a day). Because persons with dementia will often resist trying anything new, serve familiar foods whenever possible. Allow plenty of time to eat.

It is important that you call the doctor if you suspect an acute illness, depression, or a medication reaction. Analyze the particular eating problem before making any changes. Encouraging persons with dementia to maintain as much independence in eating as possible will help preserve their sense of self-esteem and reduce demands on caregivers.

Coping Strategies for Eating

Here are some suggestions to try if eating becomes a problem:

1. *Pain or problems chewing.* Have a thorough dental check of teeth, gums, and dentures.

2. *Forgetting to eat or drink fluids.* Try a telephone call, alarms, or reminder notes if the person lives alone. Hire a homemaker to prepare meals, arrange for home-delivered meals, or for attendance at a senior citizen nutrition site (see Chapter 16). Ask the doctor to monitor weight loss and evaluate malnutrition. Watch for signs of dehydration: fever, rapid pulse, flushing, confusion, dizziness, thirst.

3. *Inability to see food.* Arrange for an eye examination.

4. *Eating constantly*. Try low-calorie snacks (celery and carrot sticks or fruit), diversion to another activity such as going on a walk, or serve five or six small meals a day.

5. *Restlessness which prevents sitting down for a meal.* Offer short and frequent meals and/or nutritious snacks (cheese and crackers) that can be eaten while walking.

6. *Table manners deteriorate.* Serve meals in an area where clean-up is easiest, use a smock or apron to protect clothes, and allow plenty of time for eating.

7. *Difficulty handling utensils*. Make eating simple by providing finger foods such as sandwiches, cheese and crackers, fried chicken, fresh fruits, and vegetables.

8. *Problems chewing*. Check with the dentist to make sure dentures fit or teeth are in good repair, cut food into small pieces, or grind it.

9. *Hiding food or eating spoiled food.* If the person with dementia lives alone, spoiled food in the refrigerator or food that is improperly stored may be an indication that the living arrangement needs to be changed. Try frequent checks by family or hire a daily helper.

10. *Weight loss*. If the person with Alzheimer's disease loses more than 5 to 10 pounds in a 6-week period, consult the doctor immediately. Ask for an evaluation of physical illness, depression, or medication reactions. Nutrition supplements may be necessary.

Special Diets

Someone with multi-infarct dementia may need to restrict salt intake to control blood pressure and help prevent further strokes. Other illnesses such as diabetes may require special diets. When the person with dementia lives alone, this can be a major issue and can even be life-threatening. Controlling the food purchased at the grocery store, hiring a homemaker to prepare meals, or ordering home-delivered meals (which often provide special diets) may help (see Chapter 16), but eventually a move to a more structured living arrangement may be necessary (see Chapter 17).

Eating Out

If your relative enjoys eating in a restaurant or having a meal with family or friends, it is important to continue to provide this opportunity for socialization and stimulation.

Reduce or minimize the possibility of confusion, anxiety, or agitation by going to a restaurant at the quietest time and sharing a meal with only one or two family members or friends instead of a large group. If that does not work, try shortening the time (for example, going only for appetizers or for dessert).

If the person with Alzheimer's disease is unable to make menu choices, try reducing the number of choices by describing two selections from the menu that are favorites ("the chicken and the steak look good today; which would you prefer?").

Family or friends will probably understand poor table manners if you let them know that this behavior is part of the illness.

Eating in End-Stage Dementia

Persons in the terminal phase of a dementing illness usually have problems chewing and swallowing and may need to be fed. They are at risk for choking, which can lead to an aspiration pneumonia from a piece of food in the lung. They may resist both foods and fluids and become malnourished and dehydrated. A swallowing evaluation by a speech pathologist may be indicated. Families are faced with decisions about feeding tubes and artificial hydration. It is helpful if these issues have been addressed early in the illness and included in a power of attorney for health care (see Chapter 14). Decisions that families must make in the terminal stage are covered in Chapter 19.

Walking

Encouraging mobility is important. Regular activity and exercise during the day will promote a good night's sleep, which is essential for the person with dementia as well as the caregiver. Exercise helps maintain a regular bowel routine, and it may also decrease pacing or wandering behavior.

Activity such as walking can be included in such everyday tasks as sweeping, dusting, or raking. Many senior centers have regular exercise programs. Mall walking is popular when the weather does not invite walking outside. Exercise equipment in your home or in an exercise center can be used.

In the late stages of Alzheimer's disease or when someone with dementia has another illness such as arthritis, walking may become more difficult or even unsafe. A physical or occupational therapist (see Chapters 9 and 16) may be helpful in identifying risks, suggesting equipment, or teaching caregivers how to assist or lift without back injuries.

Because it is difficult or impossible for a person with Alzheimer's disease to relearn skills that are lost, even if they are only temporarily bedridden with an illness or injury, they may forget how to walk. Discuss with your doctor about arranging for a physical therapy evaluation as soon as it is safe for your relative to get out of bed.

In the late stages of Alzheimer's disease, walking may be so unsafe that the person is restrained to prevent falls. Restraining a person with dementia may create problems such as agitation or increased confusion. The family should discuss the risks and benefits of restraint use with the doctor.

Household Management

Household management involves a set of complex tasks that may be affected by the disease long before such habitual tasks as eating, grooming, or toileting. Household management includes meal preparation, shopping, cleaning, repairs, laundry, money management, and use of medications.

Meal Preparation

Persons with Alzheimer's disease gradually lose the ability to plan and prepare a complete meal. Early indications may include preparation of simpler meals or omission of one course. Later the person may forget to cook altogether. For a person with dementia living alone, malnutrition can result.

Home-delivered meals, meal preparation by family, hiring a homemaker (described in Chapter 16), or a change in residence are possible solutions to this problem.

If there is a caregiver in the household, try to maintain whatever skills in meal preparation are left by suggesting familiar recipes, delegating simple tasks such as chopping vegetables for soup, setting or clearing the table, or washing dishes (plastic dishes help).

Shopping

Persons with Alzheimer's disease will gradually lose the ability to shop. They may become confused by the number of choices and crowds, forget what they came to buy, be unable to make change, display large amounts of cash, or purchase items they do not need. They are vulnerable to financial abuse or exploitation if they are alone. Despite these losses, they may continue to enjoy going with someone on short shopping excursions even if they are no longer able to be completely independent.

Cleaning, Laundry, and Home Repair

Clues that laundry is not being done include soiled clothing or bedding, hiding laundry, or fewer than expected items in the laundry basket.

Even if persons with dementia can no longer initiate or follow through with the sequence of cleaning, laundry, or repairs, they may be able to perform a single task with cuing or demonstrations. Repetitious activities such as dusting, sweeping, polishing silver, or folding clothes may make them feel useful and included in the household.

Major repairs may be an unsafe activity for persons with dementia even if they have done them for years. This is particularly true when power tools are needed or when the repair could be dangerous to themselves or to others (such as trying to fix an electrical problem). Safety issues are covered in Chapter 9.

Two other household management tasks will be described in other chapters: financial management in Chapter 14 and medication use in Chapters 9 and 15.

Summary

The main message of this chapter is the need to develop realistic expectations of the person with dementia. Daily tasks are only one of many areas in which function is affected. Hygiene is another and is the subject of the next chapter.

Chapter 7

Maintaining Hygiene

Personal hygiene is the focus of this chapter. For many reasons this is often a particularly sensitive issue for the person with Alzheimer's disease as well as the family. This chapter addresses problems with bathing, grooming, toileting, and urinary and bowel incontinence.

Problems with Hygiene

Deterioration in personal hygiene is a common problem even in the early stage of a dementing illness. It is also a difficult issue for families because personal hygiene is both private and symbolic of adulthood. Not surprisingly, many persons with dementia resist any assistance with personal hygiene tasks, calling for creative strategies on the part of caregivers. Continued good personal hygiene is important for self-esteem and prevention of social isolation.

Assessment of Hygiene Tasks

As described in the last chapter, the ability to perform daily tasks can be uneven; this applies as well to hygiene. The person with dementia may continue to be meticulous about putting on lipstick or shaving every day but resist bathing. The ability to perform hygiene tasks may also vary from one day to the next.

It is important to assess each task individually. Ask whether the person is able to:

• Initiate the task independently?

- Respond to cues or demonstrations?

- Finish the task if someone else begins it?

Using bathing as an example, does the person remember to bathe at a certain time each day without a reminder? If not, would the person respond to suggestions that it is time for a bath? Or do you need to run the bath water, lay out the soap and towel, and help the person undress?

Obtain Professional Advice

Consider obtaining professional help in assessing problems with hygiene. Your doctor, nurse, or an occupational therapist (see Chapter 16) may be able to suggest other ways of handling the hygiene problems you are facing.

Independence and Self-Esteem are the Goals

With hygiene as with other daily tasks, the goal is to preserve as much independence, self-esteem, and dignity as possible without unrealistic expectations. The section in Chapter 6 on Planning Daily Activities may help to evaluate hygiene tasks.

Bathing

Bathing problems are common for persons with Alzheimer's disease. They often resist bathing, reject offers of help, and may even have a catastrophic reaction (described in Chapter 11) in response to suggestions to bathe. Causes of bathing problems can include: depression, acute illness, changed temperature sensation, fear of falling, lack of privacy, or misinterpretation of cues such as the sound of running water.

Coping Strategies for Bathing

Follow long-standing bathing habits in terms of the number of baths per week and time of day when taken. Instead of asking if they want a bath, announce the bath in a matter-of-fact manner. Offer step-by-step explanations or cues and avoid rushing. Make sure the bathroom is warm enough and maintain as much privacy as possible.

Delay bathing if the person becomes extremely agitated, anxious, or combative. Wait for a "good day," reduce the number of baths per week, or give sponge baths. Try a written order from the doctor to remind the person to bathe.

Never leave persons with Alzheimer's disease alone in the bath or shower. They may scald themselves or drown. Set the water temperature on the hot water heater at 120° to minimize the risk of scalding. Decrease the risk of falling by putting nonslip adhesive on the bottom of the tub and installing grab bars. If the person feels safer sitting down, shower benches and hand-held showers are available from medical supply stores. Consider showering with the person if it reduces anxiety.

If you are physically unable to provide assistance with bathing or if the person continues to resist bathing, enlist the help of another family member, arrange for a bath at the adult day center, or hire a bath aide (see Chapter 16). Sometimes people with Alzheimer's disease will accept help from an aide when they will not allow assistance from family members.

Grooming

Try to develop or continue a regular grooming schedule which, like bathing, closely resembles established habits. When looking at brushing teeth and care of dentures make your own assessment by asking the following questions:

- Can teeth brushing be initiated with a simple verbal cue?

- Is it necessary to help locate the bathroom and to set out the toothbrush and paste on the sink?

- Do you need to demonstrate by brushing your own teeth?

- Do you need to actually put the paste on the brush and initiate brushing?

A simple hair style is important for women. Go to a hairdresser or barber if shampooing by a professional is less frightening. It can also be a good social outing.

If you are unable to manage nail care, consider asking a nurse or podiatrist to help. Some senior centers have regularly scheduled nail care clinics for a reasonable charge.

Toileting

Like the personal hygiene tasks described earlier in this chapter, toileting is a private activity for adults. Not only is the person with dementia likely to resist assistance with toileting, but family members often feel uncomfortable offering to help.

Loss of bladder control (urinary incontinence) is common in Alzheimer's disease and may become a problem in the middle stage of the illness. Loss of bowel control (fecal incontinence), on the other hand, is less common and, if it does occur at all, usually does so late in the disease. Both urinary and bowel incontinence often begin with occasional episodes and gradually progress. Avoid criticizing the person when this happens.

Coping with incontinence is usually one of the most stressful aspects of caring for someone with Alzheimer's disease. It creates a great deal of extra physical work for the caregiver, often results in further social isolation, may be expensive, and may lead to medical complications such as breakdown of the skin. It is one of the main reasons for deciding to place someone with dementia in a nursing home. For further information on incontinence, refer to the book entitled *Coping with Bowel and Bladder Incontinence* in the *Coping with Aging Series*.

Urinary Incontinence

The following are possible contributors to urinary incontinence:

1. *Infection.* A sudden loss of bladder control may be the result of a treatable illness such as a urinary tract infection. Call the doctor immediately if this occurs.

2. *Inability to find the bathroom.* Initially this may occur in an unfamiliar place but eventually the person with Alzheimer's disease may have difficulty locating the bathroom at home. It may also occur only at night when disorientation may be more pronounced. Directions posted on the wall, a night light, or correction of vision problems may help.

3. *Inability to recognize the urge or forgetting to urinate.* Try verbal cues first ("it's time to go to the bathroom now"). If needed, take the person to the bathroom after each meal and/or every 2 to 3 hours during the day.

4. *Side effects of medications or certain fluids.* Some medications can cause or increase incontinence as can fluids such as coffee or coke. Consult the doctor.

5. *Inability to get to the toilet on time.* Although this is often related to a gradual loss of control over the nerves that control the bladder, it is made worse by either problems with mobility or a bathroom that is not readily accessible (such as upstairs). A regular toileting schedule may prevent waiting until the last minute. A urinal or a commode chair near the bed may be helpful at night if the bathroom is a distance away or if falling is a danger. See Chapter 16.

6. *Difficulty managing clothing.* The gradual loss of coordination that is a part of Alzheimer's disease often makes managing zippers, buttons, or belts difficult. Simple clothing

with an elastic waist or velcro fasteners may help (see Chapter 6 on dressing).

7. *Difficulty with balance.* Getting up and down from a regular toilet seat can be frightening to someone with balance problems. Try a raised toilet seat and/or grab bars next to the toilet (both available from medical supply stores).

8. *Difficulty communicating.* If the person with Alzheimer's disease is unable to express the need to use the toilet, you will have to become a close observer of nonverbal behavior such as increased restlessness or agitation, which may be a signal.

9. *Nighttime incontinence.* Maintain adequate fluid intake during the day to prevent dehydration (6 to 8 glasses of any fluid) but restrict fluids in the evening after dinner. Place a commode or urinal next to the bed if finding the bathroom is a problem at night.

Obtain Professional Assistance

If urinary incontinence persists, talk to your doctor or nurse. To determine any pattern to the behavior, it is helpful to keep a log of incontinence episodes. Sometimes medications can be used to help with urinary incontinence, although many of these medications have side-effects that create other problems (see Chapter 15).

Use Incontinence Products

If the urinary incontinence persists, there are many incontinence products available to help families cope. These include pads or diapers as well as pads for the bed. Your doctor or nurse can suggest which product might meet your needs. These products can be quite expensive and are usually not reimbursed by insurance. If the incontinence cannot be corrected, regular bathing becomes even more important to prevent skin breakdown.

Issues in Late Stage Alzheimer's Disease

Urinary incontinence in the later stages of Alzheimer's disease often occurs when the person is bedridden. To avoid pressure sores, the person will need to be turned to a different position regularly and will also need frequent baths. Sometimes urinary catheters can be used to catch the urine in a bag. Discuss this with your doctor.

Bowel Incontinence

The following suggestions may help prevent bowel incontinence:

- Drink 6 to 8 glasses of any fluid a day.

- Get regular exercise.

- Eat a balanced diet including plenty of fiber foods.

- Avoid over-use of laxatives.

- Maintain a regular toileting schedule (especially after each meal).

Coping with Bowel Incontinence

If bowel incontinence does occur, assess whether the factors described previously under Urinary Incontinence

·could be contributing to this problem. Monitor laxatives to prevent over-use. Some medications have either constipation or diarrhea as a side-effect. Severe constipation (fecal impaction) can sometimes cause incontinence of watery stool around hard immovable stool. If bowel incontinence persists, talk with your doctor or nurse. Ask if a fecal impaction is present.

Summary

Maintaining personal hygiene is one of the most difficult aspects of caring for someone with Alzheimer's disease. The next chapter looks at ways to encourage continued social and leisure activities.

Chapter 8

Enjoying Social and Leisure Activities

❖❖❖❖❖❖❖❖❖❖❖❖❖❖❖❖❖❖❖❖❖❖❖❖❖❖❖❖❖❖❖

Despite the illness, persons with Alzheimer's disease can continue to enjoy social and leisure activities. This chapter discusses assessing and planning appropriate activities with specific examples such as social events, hobbies, exercise, and travel.

Problems in Social and Leisure Activities

Persons with dementia gradually lose the ability to engage in social and leisure activities the way they did before their illnesses began. This change is a direct result of particular symptoms of the disease such as:

- Decreased ability to tolerate noise, confusion, or stress.

- Problems concentrating.

- Inability to follow directions, initiate activity, or learn new things.

- Recent memory loss.

- Difficulty communicating.

- Inaccurate interpretation of what is happening around them.

In addition, if they are expected to do too much or are rushed or fatigued, their performance will suffer even more.

The Importance of Social and Leisure Activities

Despite these changes, persons with Alzheimer's disease need to continue to be involved in social and leisure activities to the extent that they are able. Feeling busy and useful helps build positive self-esteem, provides companionship with others, and contributes to independence and feelings of control. Because persons with dementia are often unable to initiate activities, boredom is a common problem that can lead to other undesirable behaviors, such as wandering. Consequently, caregivers usually need to take the lead in planning recreational activities.

Assessing and Planning Activities

When looking at possible social and leisure activities, think first about what has been enjoyable for the person in the past. Starting a new activity or hobby is usually not a realistic goal. Also keep in mind that some elderly persons never had the luxury to enjoy leisure-time activities. In such instances, finding ways for them to continue to help with household tasks may be the best solution (refer to Chapter 6).

When you have a list of possible activities, ask whether the person is able to:

- Initiate the activity.

- Engage in the activity if it is suggested.

- Complete the activity if it is begun.

Take planting a garden as an example. Is your relative able to find the garden, the seeds, and the necessary tools and begin working independently? If you take him to the garden, provide instructions and tools, can he finish the task? Or do you need to work in the garden with him?

Consider Safety

The need for safety and supervision are important concerns when assessing leisure-time possibilities. Some hobbies such as woodworking or hunting may no longer be safe. If some activities are unsafe or if the supervision that is required exhausts the caregiver, the activity may need to be dropped. For a more complete discussion of safety, refer to Chapter 9.

Consider Outside Help

Many caregivers do not have the time or energy to plan, initiate, and supervise activities all day. Other members of the family, hired companions, or adult day center staff may help (see Chapter 16).

Tips on Planning Activities

Activities will have a greater chance of success if you keep the following suggestions in mind:

- Plan activities for the time of day when the person has the most energy and is the most receptive.

- Focus on what the person can do rather than on limitations. Give credit for trying rather than for completing the activity.

- Reduce distractions and avoid rushing.

- Break down activities into simple steps and provide clear instructions.

- Tailor activities to adults. People with dementia may be offended by activities they associate with children.

Just as too little activity may result in boredom, too much stimulation may lead to anxiety, confusion, disorientation, frustration, or resistance. These are clues that the activity may be too complex and should be modified or eliminated altogether.

Social Events

The ability to interact with others in social situations is frequently preserved in early dementia. Even though persons with Alzheimer's disease may not be able to completely follow conversations or may participate less, they often still enjoy the company of other people. Social activities are an important way to prevent isolation and/ or depression and to provide some stimulation. However, if there are any indications, such as restlessness, that the person is not enjoying the activity try planning activities that are shorter or that involve fewer people.

Social activities can include visits or meals with friends and family (see Chapter 6 under Eating Out for a discussion of social dining). Reminiscing can be a part of a visit and is often a satisfying activity because it draws on the person's long-term memory, which is often quite good. Old scrapbooks and pictures are a good way to prompt reminiscing.

Caregivers are sometimes embarrassed by the person's loss of social skills and as a result may withdraw from social activities. This is a time for relatives and friends to take the initiative to prevent increased isolation of both the caregiver and the person with dementia. It is also important for others to encourage the caregiver to maintain social activities, even if it means hiring a respite worker (refer to Chapter 16). Caregivers who become isolated are at risk of increased stress and possible depression (see Chapter 13).

Withdrawal by others may also occur for various reasons, including uncertainty about how to relate to the person with Alzheimer's disease, unwillingness to watch the person's deterioration, or fear that the person is crazy or the disease is contagious. Help friends understand that persons with Alzheimer's disease need contact with others, even if visits are quickly forgotten. Explain that behavior changes are part of the illness, not intentional. Prepare them for the reality that the person may not recognize them or remember their names. Help them with communication tips and suggestions for activities or assistance (see Chapter 16). Encourage short and frequent visits.

Hobbies

Because of difficulty learning new information, it is important to encourage activities that the person with Alzheimer's disease enjoyed in the past. Many of these activities can be modified to allow continued participation as the following examples illustrate:

- Listening to music might substitute for playing an instrument.

- If reading skills have been lost, consider magazines with pictures or talking books (see Chapter 16).

- Mending clothes might be satisfying even if sewing an entire outfit is no longer possible.

- Hitting golf balls can be fun even if it is not a competitive game.

- If playing bridge is frustrating, playing solitaire may still be enjoyable.

The key is to modify expectations and encourage continued activity even if the person with Alzheimer's disease is no longer performing at previous levels. As long as the person gets some satisfaction or enjoyment from the activity, it serves its purpose.

Exercise

Regular exercise has many benefits. It can help calm someone who is anxious or restless. It can promote a good night's sleep and prevent constipation. It can decrease isolation by offering an opportunity to be with other people. It does not call on the person with Alzheimer's disease to think.

A daily walk (outside or in a mall), group exercise classes (often offered in senior centers), or participation in a fitness center program are good ways to get exercise. Check with the doctor before beginning a new exercise program.

Traveling

The ability of a person with Alzheimer's disease to enjoy or tolerate travel will decline as the disease progresses. Trial and error is the only way for families to learn whether traveling can be tolerated or enjoyed at each stage. It may not be a good idea if it offers too much stimulation, activity, or pressure or if it results in increased disorientation. What worked 6 months ago may not work now. An increase in anxiety, irritability, fatigue, confusion, or wandering may be cues that traveling is becoming more difficult.

Here are some suggestions for simplifying traveling:

- Go on a tour (eliminates driving, concerns about schedules, tickets, and baggage).

- Go somewhere and stay an extended period rather than changing location frequently.

- If you are visiting with a group, try to find a quiet spot and time for resting.

- When overnight traveling becomes too difficult, try day trips to familiar places.

- If an all-day trip is too taxing, go for a short ride in the car.

If you do travel with someone with dementia, maintain the daily routine as closely as possible, especially meals, bedtime, and rest periods. Allow plenty of time for everyday tasks. Make sure the person with Alzheimer's disease has identification such as the name of the hotel. Relatives should take responsibility for most of the money and important papers such as tickets and passports. Bring a night light. Try frequent toileting to reduce accidents. Public restrooms are often a problem if the person with Alzheimer's disease relies on the spouse for help in toileting. One solution is to invite a companion of the same sex who can accompany the person into public restrooms.

Escort service from the airlines can be arranged for someone with early dementia who may become confused changing planes. A person with mid to late stage dementia should never travel alone. When traveling is no longer appropriate for someone with Alzheimer's disease, caregivers who enjoy traveling should arrange for respite care (see Chapters 16 and 17) so that they can look forward to continued trips.

Summary

The previous three chapters have focused on how Alzheimer's disease affects all aspects of everyday life. It also has a major impact on safety, which is the subject of the next chapter.

Chapter 9

Safety

This chapter discusses safety, which is almost always a major concern for caregivers of persons with Alzheimer's disease. It describes how the illness affects safety, how dangerous situations can be prevented, and how to cope with common safety problems such as driving, drugs and alcohol, fires, falling, getting lost, emergencies, and living alone. Finally, it provides suggestions for assessing safety risks and deciding how and when to intervene.

Safety: A Common Problem

Unlike most other illnesses, Alzheimer's disease inevitably results in concerns about safety. Even before the diagnosis is made, unsafe behavior may become apparent and may be one reason for seeking a medical evaluation. Persons with dementia are often unaware of safety risks posed by their behavior and may retain good social skills that obscure safety problems. Because their abilities may decline at an uneven rate, some activities may continue to be safe while others may become dangerous.

Unsafe Behavior: A Result of the Disease

Unsafe behavior is a direct consequence of a dementing illness. Because Alzheimer's disease impairs short-term memory, it becomes increasingly difficult to remember when to turn off the stove burner, how to use a traffic light to cross a busy street, or how to call for help in an emergency. Because Alzheimer's disease affects judgment, the person will no longer be able to evaluate whether a given situation is safe or dangerous, assess consequences, and decide what action is required. Because Alzheimer's disease interferes with concentration, the person may be easily distracted from a task such as driving, which requires complete attention. Because Alzheimer's disease eventually results in changes in coordination, reaction time and balance gradually become impaired.

Safety: A Difficult Problem for Caregivers

Because persons with Alzheimer's disease often are unaware of the changes caused by the illness, they may strongly resist any attempts on the part of family or others to restrict their independence in the interest of safety. Reactions such as anger, defiance, frustration, and depression are common.

For families, safety is one of the most difficult problems posed by a progressive dementing illness. It requires that caregivers become astute observers of all activities. They learn they can no longer defer to the judgment of the person with dementia about what is safe but must instead rely on their own judgments. Almost all families eventually decide they must limit certain activities.

No one wants to accept that someone they love is deteriorating. Few family members are comfortable restricting the activities of an adult relative. Many caregivers have little energy or time to assume the burden of extra tasks that the person with Alzheimer's disease can no longer safely perform. Many families find it difficult to objectively evaluate which activities are still safe and which are dangerous. Nevertheless, because unsafe behaviors can cause serious harm or even death to the person with

Alzheimer's disease or others, caregivers need to deal with safety before a tragedy occurs.

Prevention of Safety Problems

The best way to deal with potential threats to safety is prevention. This involves creating calm and safe surroundings to reduce potential hazards. The role of the surroundings in Alzheimer's disease cannot be overemphasized. Persons with dementia gradually lose the ability to understand and respond appropriately to their surroundings. They have difficulty screening out stimulation that they once ignored. For example, a busy pattern in a rug or a mirror may suddenly cause anxiety or confusion. Difficulty interpreting external stimulation is common. For example, when persons with Alzheimer's disease become agitated by violence on television, they probably fear that the violence is occurring right in their own homes.

Caregivers need to carefully observe what things in the surroundings contribute to increased confusion, anxiety, or agitation and take steps to simplify the home. However, this does not mean eliminating all stimulation or making so many simultaneous changes that the home becomes unrecognizable.

A Calm Home is Important

When persons with dementia become anxious, confused or agitated, they are less predictable and at greater risk of engaging in unsafe activity. For example, someone who is agitated may flee into a busy street. Accidents such as falls are more likely to occur when the person with dementia is hurried or pressured. The mood of the caregiver is also an important factor in the creation of a calm atmosphere.

Tips on Creating a Calm Home

Some of the following suggestions for changes in the home or schedule may reduce confusion or behavior problems.

- Reduce background noise such as a radio or television. This may lessen confusion or anxiety and also increase the ability to concentrate.

- Limit the number of activities or visitors if they are causing fatigue or agitation.

- Allow plenty of time to engage in everyday tasks without rushing. This may mean that to get to the doctor's appointment on time you need to begin to get ready 2 hours beforehand.

- Simplify the living areas of the home if too much clutter is confusing.

Tips on Creating a Safe Home

Persons with Alzheimer's disease and other dementias are prone to accidents. Although elimination of all risk is never possible, trying to prevent accidents by creating a safe home is worthwhile. The steps you take to prevent accidents will vary with the stage of the illness and what you anticipate as the major risks. You will need to carefully evaluate and reevaluate the capacities and limits of the person with dementia as the illness progresses. In the early stages of a dementing illness, driving, becoming lost, and the inability to manage medications may be the major safety risks. Later, fires and falls may become the main hazards.

The first step in creating safe surroundings is to systematically assess the home, looking for ways to prevent falls, fires, poisoning, and accidents. The following section of this chapter describes both what to look for and possible solutions for major safety hazards. If you need professional help with a general safety evaluation, arrange for a visit from an occupational therapist or nurse from one of the home health agencies in your community (refer to Chapter 16).

If you decide to do your own safety assessment, here are some suggestions of potentially dangerous items to look for and lock up or remove if necessary:

- Sharp or dangerous kitchen utensils such as knives, food processors, mixers, toaster ovens, coffee makers.

- Outside equipment including lawn mowers, chainsaws, snowblowers, gasoline containers, ladders, boats, farm implements.

- Weapons, especially guns.

- Items in the basement such as electric power tools or paint.

- Poisons such as cleaning supplies, insecticides, or poisonous plants.

- Alcohol and drugs.

- Objects that might be eaten such as buttons, pins, or wax fruit.

Driving

Regardless of the stage of the illness, research has shown that people with Alzheimer's disease are at high risk of having or causing driving accidents. Unsafe driving is a danger not only to the person with dementia but to the general public. Most experts recommend not driving as soon as the diagnosis is established.

Driving is an extremely complex task that is affected by the following symptoms of dementia: memory loss, impaired judgment, disorientation, slowed reaction time, inability to make decisions, poor coordination, and decreased alertness. All of these symptoms will only get worse as the illness progresses. In addition, vision and hearing loss or the use of sedating medications or alcohol can make driving even less safe.

Recognizing Unsafe Driving

The following are all clues that driving is no longer a safe activity:

- Getting lost.

- Driving too fast or too slow.

- Not staying in the proper lane or making inappropriate lane changes.

- Making wide right turns.

- Not stopping completely at stop signs.

- Angry or aggressive driving.

- Causing or being involved in an accident.

- Needing cues from passengers.

Some think that persons with dementia may be safe if they drive only in familiar neighborhoods and/or if someone is with them to provide instructions. However, even in a familiar neighborhood the unexpected can occur, such as a child running in front of the car. Persons with Alzheimer's disease cannot be counted on to respond appropriately in a crisis because they are unable to quickly interpret multiple stimuli, make appropriate decisions, and respond instantaneously, even with directions from others.

Resistance to Driving Limits

Driving in our culture is both a symbol of adulthood and a means of maintaining independence and control over one's life. Because persons with Alzheimer's disease are usually unaware of their driving problems, they are often unwilling to voluntarily give up driving. They also may not be able to understand that continued driving may threaten the financial security of their family because of liability. Caregivers who permit continued unsafe driving may also be held liable if there is an accident and a lawsuit.

Coping with Unsafe Driving

Here are some suggestions for ways to limit unsafe driving:

- At the time of the diagnosis, ask the physician to address the driving issue directly with both the person with dementia and the family so everyone will know exactly what was said.

- A written recommendation from the doctor may be helpful later if the person with Alzheimer's disease forgets the conversation.

- If needed, enlist the help of others who are influential (another family member, clergy, lawyer, insurance agent, or law enforcement officer) to persuade the person with dementia to voluntarily give up driving.

- Use the financial argument, including the possibility of liability after an accident or the increased cost of insurance.

- If voluntary compliance is resisted, discuss with the doctor the possibility of notifying the state motor vehicle department or licensing agency. Families can also contact the appropriate state agency directly. Each state has different regulations regarding who can report unsafe drivers, whether the reports are confidential, and what steps the state can take to limit driving.

- Sell or remove the car if the person with dementia is the only driver in the household.

- Hide the car keys.

- If there is a spouse who is a nondriver, encourage driving lessons.

- If no one in the household drives, explore other means of transportation in the community (refer to Chapter 16).

Drugs and Alcohol

People with dementing illnesses frequently have problems taking medications correctly. These problems are a direct result of the dementia, especially changes in memory, orientation, and judgment.

Problems with medications include both prescription as well as nonprescription medications (known as over-the-counter drugs). Sometimes the inability to handle medications is obvious, and sometimes it is subtle and more difficult for families to assess.

Alcohol is also a drug. Persons with dementia who have a history of overuse of alcohol will probably continue this pattern.

Why Drug Misuse is Dangerous

In general, older people consume a disproportionate amount of medications, and persons with Alzheimer's disease are no exception. In addition to a dementia, they often suffer from other chronic illnesses such as arthritis, diabetes, or high blood pressure for which they are taking medications. All drugs, whether they are prescription or over-the-counter, have risks; the more medications one takes the higher the risk of adverse reactions. In addition, as people age, their bodies tolerate medications less well, and they may need to have the dose adjusted downward.

Why Alcohol Use is Dangerous

As people age, their bodies have less tolerance for alcohol. Even small amounts of alcohol in a healthy older person may seriously interfere with physical coordination and the ability to think clearly and make good judgments. Use of alcohol in any amount by someone with dementia compounds confusion, disorientation, and risks of a serious accident.

Recognizing Medication Misuse

Watch for both overuse and underuse of medications resulting from short-term memory loss or disorientation. Persons who cannot remember what they did 5 minutes ago can easily forget that they already took their medications and take more. Confusion about time or day of the week will complicate following a medication schedule accurately.

Be aware of the possibility of hoarding, hiding, or throwing out drugs, which is often done secretly and frequently results from suspicion about medications.

Look at whether the person with dementia is taking expired medications or drugs prescribed for another member of the household.

Investigate whether prescriptions are being obtained from several different physicians or pharmacies.

Watch for sudden changes in mental status such as acute confusion, sedation, or hallucinations, which might indicate a delirium caused by drugs (refer to Chapter 3).

Medication Abuse

Medication abuse (use of illegal drugs or addiction to prescription drugs) is another possible problem that may have started long before the diagnosis of dementia. The most widely abused drugs are: sedative-hypnotics (such as sleeping pills), narcotics (including pain pills), benzodiazepines ("nerve" pills), over-the-counter pain medications, antidepressants, and antihistamines (cough and cold medications). If you notice excessive use of any of these drugs, consult the doctor at once.

Recognizing Alcohol Problems

Most persons who drink alcohol in excess minimize or deny the problem. Someone with a dementia may be unable to remember how much alcohol has been consumed. Caregivers need to watch for concrete evidence of alcohol use, such as finding hidden alcohol bottles in the house, empty bottles in the trash, or reports of frequent purchases by a local liquor store.

Other signs of alcohol use are harder to assess because they may also be symptoms of dementia. They include:

falls, diarrhea, urinary incontinence, dramatic mood swings, confusion and memory loss, self-neglect, malnutrition, and isolation.

Coping with Medication Misuse

Discuss your concerns with the physician or nurse. Try to simplify the medication schedule so that all medications are taken only once or twice a day.

If there is more that one doctor prescribing medications, make sure they are all aware of what medications are being used. Take all medications (prescription and over-the-counter) to all doctor's appointments.

Put medications in a daily or weekly pill box (available in most drug stores) and monitor carefully. Remove the pill bottle to prevent extra medications from being taken.

Arrange for a visiting nurse to set up and monitor medications once a week (refer to Chapter 16). This service will probably not be reimbursed by Medicare except for a brief period after an acute illness. Day care center staff can usually dispense medications.

Call at a prearranged time to remind the person with Alzheimer's disease to take the medications or purchase a medication box with an alarm that will go off when it is time to take the pill. This will no longer work when the person with dementia forgets what the alarm means.

Use only one pharmacy in order to monitor overuse or underuse of a given medication or misuse of over-the-counter drugs. Throw out all out-dated medications and lock up medications if necessary.

If the person refuses to take an essential medication, it can be crushed and hidden in food only after all other alternatives have been exhausted.

Keep a log book of medication names, doses, possible side effects, the purpose of each medication, and the dates begun or stopped.

Coping with Alcohol Abuse

Because it is unlikely that anyone with a dementing illness will be able to benefit from an alcohol treatment program, the focus needs to be on increasing the amount of supervision and structure in order to eliminate the use of alcohol. This is difficult if the person with dementia lives alone, and it could involve attendance at an adult day center or hiring aides. It might also be possible to cut off the supply of alcohol by talking to the liquor store personnel or restricting funds. Sometimes, moving the person to a residential facility (described in Chapter 17) is the only option.

Fires

The main risks of fire are unsafe use of the stove and careless smoking. Both problems stem primarily from loss of short-term memory and poor judgment. Because a fire can cause injury or death to others in addition to the person with dementia, the risk of fire should be carefully assessed. In the event of a fire it should not be assumed that a person with Alzheimer's disease will have the judgment to respond appropriately.

Recognizing Fire Hazards

Here are some clues that there is a risk for fire:

- Stove burners left on.

- Scorched or burned pots or food.

- Cigarette burns on the person, clothes, furniture, carpet, or floor.

- Cigarette butts hidden throughout the house.

Coping with Fire Hazards

Here are some suggestions for preventing a fire:

- Make sure there is a smoke alarm that works. If possible, connect it to the apartment office or fire station so that someone in addition to the person with dementia will be alerted if it goes off.

- Explore the possibility of a microwave. If the person with Alzheimer's disease already knows how to operate a microwave or can learn to do so, remove the knobs of the regular stove or disconnect it.

- Limit the amount of cooking by bringing in prepared meals, hiring a homemaker, or arranging for home-delivered meals (see Chapter 16).

- Explore the possibility of a timer on an electric stove that will automatically shut off after a specified length of time.

- Call the local fire department to see whether there is a program for registering persons with disabilities so that in case of a fire they will be rescued first.

- Allow smoking only in one area and only with supervision. Lock up all smoking material when not in use.

Falling

Falling is an increasingly frequent problem as people age. Falling can cause serious injuries, such as hip fractures, and is a common reason for admissions to hospitals and nursing homes. Persons with Alzheimer's disease are at even greater risk of falling than the general population because of disorientation, poor judgment, and loss of coordination. For example, lack of judgment may lead someone with dementia to climb an unsafe ladder. In the later stage of the disease, loss of coordination may include poor balance and/or an abnormal gait.

Fall Prevention

Because falls are potentially so disabling, prevention is important. The first step in fall prevention is to assess the home and make whatever changes are needed. Pay particular attention to the bathroom and to stairs, which are the sites of most falls. Here are some ideas for preventing falls:

- Use nonskid wax on vinyl floors.

- Remove any throw rugs or fasten them to the floor.

- Use nonskid surfaces such as textured strips or decals in the bathtub or shower.

- Install grab bars near the toilet and in the bath. Consider a raised toilet seat, shower stool, and a hand-held shower (refer to Chapter 16).

- Make sure hallways and stairways are well lit and free of clutter.

- Use a nightlight in the bedroom and/or bathroom.

- Install secure railings on all stairs and mark the edges of stairs with brightly colored tape. Install gates on the top of stairs if needed.

- Remove any tripping hazards such as extension cords.

- Encourage the use of sturdy chairs that have high seats and strong arms.

- Make sure the person with dementia wears shoes that are comfortable and safe.

- Correct or treat other health problems that may increase the risk of falling, such as hearing and vision loss or arthritis.

- Closely monitor medication use, especially those that could cause dizziness or confusion. Check with the doctor immediately if you suspect a medication reaction (see Chapter 15).

- Consider the use of an emergency alarm to alert others if there is a fall (refer to Chapter 16).

Coping with a Fall

If you are with the person who has Alzheimer's disease when a fall occurs, call the emergency number to summon the rescue squad or ambulance if the person is unconscious, bleeding, or in great pain. If the person is conscious and does not seem to be in pain, summon someone else to assist you with lifting so that you do not injure yourself also.

After a fall it is important to observe carefully for any marked change in function or alertness. Persons with Alzheimer's disease are often unable to describe symptoms of pain. If you notice any change after a fall, contact the doctor.

Getting Lost

Disorientation and decreased short-term memory can result in getting lost. Often this first occurs in unfamiliar places, but later in the illness persons with Alzheimer's disease may get lost in their own neighborhoods or even in their own homes. Sometimes this occurs more frequently at night and may be part of "sundowning" behavior (described in Chapter 11). Wherever it occurs, it is a major worry for families, and it is usually a clue that more supervision is needed.

Getting lost is a concern because persons with a dementing illness are at major risk for pedestrian accidents, exposure to extreme weather conditions, or mugging. Despite these risks, however, the benefits of being allowed to walk alone to a nearby store or around the block may outweigh the possible problems created by getting lost.

You should, however, make sure the person with Alzheimer's disease wears an ID bracelet or other identification when going out. You can order a "Medic Alert" bracelet or necklace by calling 1-800-432-5378. A local jewelry store may be able to engrave an ID.

Coping with Getting Lost

Getting lost is often a result of wandering, the causes and prevention of which are described in Chapter 11.

It is a good idea to alert your neighbors and the local police to the possible risk of getting lost. Some communities have programs that register persons who are confused or disoriented. Check with the police department or the Alzheimer's Association. Even if there is no such program in your area, you can provide the police with a recent photograph. If the person with Alzheimer's disease does get lost, notify the police right away and ask that they begin a search immediately rather than waiting the customary 24 hours. Alert the emergency room at your local hospital and remain by the phone.

Emergencies

Regardless of age or health status, we are all at risk for sudden illness or injury. As described earlier in this chapter, persons with Alzheimer's disease are at greater risk. How to cope with various emergencies that may befall the person with dementia are covered in other chapters including illnesses and injuries (Chapter 15) and victimization (Chapter 14).

Plan Ahead for Caregiver Emergencies

Because it is usually unsafe to leave a person with advanced Alzheimer's disease alone for even a short period of time, the sudden unavailability of the primary caregiver requires that someone else immediately assume responsibility for the care of the person with dementia. It is best to be prepared for this possibility before it happens. Here are some ideas:

- Make arrangements for others to assume care at a moment's notice: family, friend, neighbor, home health care agency offering 24-hour care, group home, or nursing home. Make sure your family or others know what arrangements you have made and what they need to do.

- Post emergency information in a prominent place such as the refrigerator door or next to the phone. Include:

  Family names, addresses, work and home phone numbers. Indicate whom to contact in an emergency and whom you have selected to make health care decisions for you if you are incapacitated (refer to Chapter 14).

  A statement that the person you care for has Alzheimer's disease or another dementing illness and cannot be left alone even briefly.

Neighbors and friends and their phone numbers.

Doctor's name and phone number, including the number for weekends and evenings.

Name and address of preferred hospital.

Insurance names and policy numbers.

Lists of medications, schedules, and where they are kept for both the person with Alzheimer's disease and the caregiver.

Enter emergency phone numbers such as police, fire, ambulance, doctor, and emergency room in an automatic dial phone and mark in red. Eventually, however, the person with Alzheimer's disease probably will no longer be able to use a phone to summon help in a crisis. Daily checks by family or neighbors may be the only option if the caregiver's health is fragile.

Living Alone

It is obvious that people with Alzheimer's disease are safer if they are supervised than if they either live alone or are alone for significant periods of time when their caregivers are at work. In addition to all the safety hazards described earlier, a person with dementia who is alone may forget to eat or take medications, may invite strangers into the home, or may be unable to summon help if needed.

The community services described in Chapter 16 can be used to increase the supervision and safety of someone with Alzheimer's disease who is alone. Moving in with relatives or entering a residential facility or nursing home are all options that are covered in Chapters 13, 17, and 18. In cases of extreme self-neglect, it may be necessary to take legal steps such as guardianship and/or placement in a protected living situation (see Chapter 14).

When and How to Intervene

Deciding whether to intervene if there are risks to safety is one of the most difficult dilemmas faced by caregivers of persons with dementing illnesses.

Families May Not Agree

The first part of this chapter provided clues for assessing the risks of unsafe driving, fires, falls, getting lost, and living alone. The difficulty in such assessments is that often everyone in the family has a somewhat different interpretation of safety problems as well as a different tolerance for risk. Some people in the family may feel strongly that the person with Alzheimer's disease should remain independent in spite of obvious risks to safety, but others may feel equally strongly that safety is more important than preserving independence. Some may be unable to face the reality that there are safety issues at all, while others will be aware of these problems. These differences in view often lead to conflict, discomfort, or anxiety within the family.

No Right Answers

Unfortunately, there is no formula that can be used in every situation to resolve differences and arrive at an acceptable plan. Any decision that is made will carry its own risk. It is never possible to anticipate all the consequences of even the most well thought out plan. For example, if a family insists that a person with Alzheimer's disease move to a supervised living setting, the risk of accidents may decrease but the risk of greater disorientation or severe depression may increase. Use of restraints in a nursing home may prevent a fall but at the same time may increase the risk of agitated behavior or pressure sores.

Harm to Innocent Persons

When looking at unsafe behavior, the risk of injury or death to innocent victims needs to be taken into account. Unsafe driving and fires pose the greatest threat to others. Caregivers need to ask themselves how they would feel if their inaction or indecision resulted not only in harm to the person with Alzheimer's disease but to others.

Enlist Outside Help

A fresh look at your situation by an experienced professional may help both in objectively assessing risks and in deciding how and when to intervene. Possible sources of help include your doctor, nurse, social worker, case manager, visiting nurse, or occupational therapist. Support groups (often sponsored by the local Alzheimer's Association) will almost always include family caregivers who have struggled with similar issues and whose solutions might work in your situation (see Chapter 16). In the end, however, it is your decision as the caregiver.

Neither a professional nor the person with Alzheimer's disease who is no longer able to recognize safety risks can take the necessary steps to assure safety.

Summary

Safety issues are an inevitable part of a progressive illness such as Alzheimer's disease and force difficult decisions about restricting independence. These issues are even more complicated for families because the person with Alzheimer's disease often is unable to recognize safety risks and is resistant to any limits imposed by others. Another challenge for families is the emotional changes that come with the disease. This is the subject of the next chapter.

Chapter 10

Emotional Changes

Some persons who are diagnosed with a dementia exhibit changes in emotion that are difficult for families to understand and manage. This chapter will discuss why such change occurs and how to cope. It focuses on the most common emotions: depression, anxiety, frustration, anger, and suspicion.

Understanding Emotional Changes

Imagine that you have been transported to another world where nothing looks familiar, you are unable to understand either written or verbal communication, and you cannot make yourself understood. Persons with Alzheimer's disease frequently find themselves in such an unfamiliar world. They do not always recognize the people in it, and the people behave in ways that are incomprehensible or frightening. It is difficult to perform even the simplest task and communicating with others is frustrating. Although not all people with a dementing illness exhibit changes in emotion, many do express feelings of depression, anxiety, frustration, anger, or suspicion. They may also experience fear and helplessness. These feelings may be subtle and/or temporary, or they may become pervasive and difficult for families to manage. They may change as the illness progresses.

Explore Reversible Causes

If a sudden change in emotion occurs, it is important to call the doctor who can look for any reversible medical causes such as the following:

• Delirium (see Chapter 3).

- Acute illness or injury (refer to Chapter 15).

- Side-effects of medications (see Chapter 15).

Next, families should look at other external factors that might influence mood such as: stress, fatigue, excessive demands, change in routine, too many activities, or too little stimulation. For example, if the level of anxiety tends to increase in the late afternoon, is fatigue a factor? If so, see what happens if a nap is scheduled. If irritability is a problem, is it caused by the inability to initiate any activity? Would an adult day care program alleviate boredom? As these examples imply, experimenting with one small change at a time is the key.

Alzheimer's Causes Change in Emotions

Brain damage brought about by the dementing illness often leads to loss of emotional control or an inability to express emotions in socially acceptable ways. Because it is a consequence of the dementia, it cannot be reversed, and it is not deliberate. Rather than taking it personally, blame the illness instead of the person.

Depression

In 1989 the National Institute of Mental Health estimated that over 10 percent of the elderly living in the community exhibit symptoms of depression. Depression is not a normal consequence of aging; it can occur in persons already diagnosed with Alzheimer's disease or other dementias. When persons with dementing illnesses also suffer from clinical depression, their intellectual abilities decline even further. Depression is usually a treatable illness and if the depression responds to treatment, the person with dementia will have a better quality of life and will be better able to cope with losses caused by the dementia. It is therefore important for caregivers to watch for signs of depression.

Diagnosis of Depression

The diagnosis of depression needs to be made by a medical doctor or a mental health professional such as a psychiatrist or clinical psychologist. The symptoms of depression include:

- Physical changes such as decreased energy, change in appetite, altered sleep pattern, and aches and pains that do not improve with treatment.

- Mood changes such as pervasive sadness, feeling empty or bored, hopeless or helpless, poor self-esteem, anxiety, loss of interest or pleasure in activities, and thoughts of death or suicide.

- Behavior changes such as withdrawal, restlessness, irritability, difficulty concentrating or remembering, neglect of appearance or other responsibilities, and frequent tearfulness.

The diagnosis of depression in someone who already has a dementing illness is difficult to make, because the person may not be able to remember the symptoms and because many of the symptoms of dementia and depression are similar. In addition, symptoms of depression are often ignored or viewed as normal sadness. Professionals who are assessing depression need to rely heavily on the observations of family or other caregivers who are in frequent contact with the person.

The Risk of Suicide

The diagnosis of depression is important not only for reasons of quality of life but also because, without proper treatment, depression can be life-threatening. It can lead to malnutrition, self-neglect, or suicide. According to the National Institute of Mental Health (1991), the highest rates of suicide are among persons over age 65, the same group most likely to have a dementing illness. In terms of Alzheimer's disease, the risk of suicide is greatest in the early stages of the illness simply because most persons with mid to late Alzheimer's disease lack the ability to make and carry out a suicide plan. Although there is always some risk of suicide at the time of diagnosis of any terminal illness, the majority of terminally ill persons do not choose to end their lives. Those who do almost always suffer from a clinical depression which, if treated, may change their minds about suicide.

Clues that someone is considering suicide include the symptoms of depression described previously plus remarks about death or suicide, giving away possessions, changing a will, or making funeral arrangements. If you suspect the possibility of suicide, contact your doctor immediately and remain with the person until an evaluation can be made.

Treatment of Depression

Most persons suffering from depression respond positively to treatment. Treatment options can include some or all of the following approaches:

- Antidepressant medications administered by a medical doctor or a psychiatrist (discussed in Chapter 15).

- Individual counseling by a psychiatrist, psychologist, psychiatric nurse, or social worker.

- Group counseling. Although most support groups sponsored by local chapters of the Alzheimer's Association or other agencies are for caregivers, there are sometimes support groups designed specifically for persons in the early stages of dementing illnesses.

- Changes in the environment that decrease social isolation and withdrawal. Examples would include attendance at an adult day center or friendly visitors (see Chapter 16).

Anxiety

Anxiety is another signal that something is wrong. For persons with Alzheimer's disease, anxiety is frequently present and can be the result of any number of factors such as:

- Short-term memory loss including the inability to recognize familiar people, places, or things.

- The inability to express needs and/or to understand what others are saying.

- Fear of doing something wrong.

- Boredom on the one hand or too much stimulation on the other.

- Depression.

- Need for safety, comfort, or security.

- Side-effects of medications.

Anxiety can be expressed in a variety of ways such as fidgeting, pacing, inability to sit still, repetitive questions, or frequent phone calls to family or police at all hours. Coping with anxiety is stressful for families or other caregivers.

Treatment of Anxiety

As described in the beginning of this chapter, reversible causes of anxiety need to be assessed. Because anxiety is frequently seen in association with depression, an evaluation of depression should be discussed with the doctor. Sometimes medications are helpful in alleviating or controlling anxiety, although side-effects such as an increased risk of falling must be carefully weighed (see Chapter 15).

Other suggestions for coping with anxiety include:

- Reducing distractions or activities when fatigue is greatest.

- Channeling the anxiety into constructive activity such as going for a walk.

- Providing reassurance.

- Providing greater structure for persons living alone such as hiring aides to come in regularly, sending them to an adult day care program (see Chapter 16), or moving them to a residential facility (refer to Chapter 17).

- Nonverbal expressions of caring and security, such as holding hands and giving hugs.

Trying to reason with a person with anxiety is almost always futile and may only make the anxiety worse.

Frustration and Anger

It is not surprising that persons with Alzheimer's disease exhibit frustration or anger in the face of the losses they are experiencing every day. It is easier to be understanding of frustration than anger because we can all imagine how we would feel if we had difficulty performing even the simplest everyday task. Anger, however, is much less easy to understand, especially when it takes the form of socially unacceptable behavior such as yelling, throwing, or even hitting and when it is directed at the persons who are attempting to provide care. It is easier to tolerate if it is seen as an extension of extreme frustration or fear. It is almost always a direct result of the illness over which the person has no control.

Because the anger is not controllable, however, does not mean that physical abuse should be tolerated. If the person you are caring for becomes dangerous, contact your doctor or the police at once. You have a right to safety.

As with other emotional changes, the causes of frustration and anger need to be explored. Sometimes you will find an obvious connection between an activity and frustration, such as unsuccessfully trying to balance a checkbook. Anger is often triggered by frightening tasks such as bathing. Both frustration and anger, however, can also appear without warning and with no apparent connection to an external event. These unpredictable outbursts can be frightening for families and can have other serious consequences, such as discharge from an adult day care program or home care services. Keep careful records of angry outbursts and discuss them with your doctor. In some instances, medication may be helpful (see Chapter 15).

Here are some ways to cope with frustration or anger:

- Whenever possible, try to prevent frustration or anger from building up. Maintaining a calm home and having realistic expectations are both key preventive measures (see Chapter 9 for more information).

- When frustration is frequent, look for ways to encourage tasks that will be successful and build self-esteem (see Chapters 6 and 8).

- If possible, postpone activities that cause frustration and anger until the person is having a better day.

- Use the short-term memory loss to your advantage by changing the focus to a less frustrating or anxiety-producing activity or conversation. The person with dementia may very quickly forget what was upsetting.

- Provide reassurance either verbally or through nonverbal behavior.

- Call for help immediately if the behavior becomes dangerous.

Do not argue. It usually only increases anger or frustration.

Suspicion

Expressing suspicion of others is a frequent occurrence in persons with Alzheimer's disease. Often it takes the form of accusing someone else of stealing things that are misplaced, lost, or hidden. From the point of view of someone with dementia, it is a logical conclusion. The wallet has vanished at the same time a relative is visiting; therefore, the relative took the wallet. It is a way of preserving self-esteem, explaining otherwise bewildering events, and trying desperately to maintain some control. It is a direct result of the dementia including memory loss, anxiety, inability to recognize familiar people and places, or even hallucinations (seeing or hearing things that are not there, described in Chapter 11). Families need to look at suspicion as an expression of the illness instead of a deliberate character attack.

Suggestions for Coping with a Suspicious Person

Here are some ideas for managing suspicion:

- Assess whether vision or hearing problems or too much stimulation could be leading to misinterpretation of external events.

- Respond with reassurance to the underlying fear and anxiety about a world that no longer makes sense to the person with dementia.

- Discuss this behavior with your doctor. If the person becomes so suspicious that it interferes with care, there may be medication that will help (refer to Chapter 15). There also may be some reversible medical reason such as an acute illness or reactions to medications.

- Share your experience with others in a support group. You will find you are not alone, and you may come away with coping strategies that have worked for others.

- Try using diversion to shift the focus away from accusations.

- Avoid arguing or confronting, which usually only makes matters worse.

- Explain to agency staff that these accusations are a result of the illness.

People who have Alzheimer's disease or another de-menting illness are vulnerable to financial or physical abuse. There are occasions when their suspicions may be well-founded and should not be dismissed simply as symptoms of the disease. If you suspect abuse of any kind, contact your doctor, lawyer, the local Alzheimer's Association, or your local office on aging for advice about the laws in your state and what measures are available to protect the person who is ill (refer to Chapters 13 and 14).

Summary

It is important to be alert to change in emotions, some of which may be treatable while others may be an inevitable part of the disease process. Alzheimer's disease not only causes changes in emotions but also changes in behavior, which are addressed in the next chapter.

References

National Institute of Mental Health. (1989). Fact Sheet: *Depression in the elderly.*
National Institute of Mental Health. (1991). Fact Sheet: *Suicide in the elderly.*

Chapter 11

Behavioral Changes

The focus of this chapter is on the behavioral changes that accompany a dementing illness and which are often stressful for families. The chapter begins with an overview of the causes of behavior change in dementia and then covers strategies for assessment, prevention, and management. It concludes with a description of specific challenging behaviors such as: repetitive questions, losing and hiding things, withdrawal, stubbornness, sleep disturbances, "sundowning," wandering, agitation and aggression, antisocial acts, and hallucinations and delusions.

Why Change in Behavior Occurs

Although all persons with Alzheimer's disease or other dementing illnesses inevitably exhibit behavioral changes, some may be relatively minor and easy for families to tolerate while others may cause extreme exhaustion or even danger to caregivers. It is these latter behaviors that pose the most difficult challenge and which may cause community agencies to discontinue service or may result in nursing home placement.

Behavior Change is not Deliberate

The main thing for families to keep in mind is that change in behavior is a symptom of the brain disease. This means that the behavior change is not something the person with dementia can control. Knowing that it is not intentional may help families to avoid blaming the person in their care.

Because the behavior often fluctuates from day to day, it is sometimes interpreted to mean that the person with

Alzheimer's disease has more control over behavior than is actually the case. The deterioration caused by the disease is uneven so there will be good days and bad days. Some behaviors such as social skills can remain intact until late in the illness whereas other behaviors such as wandering can appear early. This unpredictability is a major source of stress for caregivers who have no idea what tomorrow will bring.

Behavior Change Caused by the Disease

Certain symptoms of Alzheimer's disease contribute directly to the change in behavior that occurs. They may include a decrease in the ability to:

- Tolerate noise, confusion, or stress.

- Concentrate.

- Express feelings, ideas, or needs.

- Follow directions.

- Perform everyday tasks.

- Recognize danger.

- Interpret events accurately.

- Solve problems.

- Initiate activities.

- Understand what others are saying.

- Remember recent events.

All of these symptoms lead to frequent feelings of fear, anger, frustration, confusion, and insecurity which, in turn, can cause behavior change. For example, boredom often occurs when initiating activities is no longer possible. When people who have dementia are bored, it may be expressed by such behaviors as wandering or withdrawing.

Other Causes of Behavior Change

In addition to symptoms of the illness described above, some behavior can result from:

- Being rushed.

- Being fatigued.

- Having other acute illnesses or injuries.

- Reacting to medications.

- Responding to the moods of other people.

- Being asked to do too many things at one time.

Coping with Behavior Change

The goal in coping with behavior change is not to alter the course of the disease but to manage the behavior so it causes the least possible distress to both the person with dementia and the caregiver.

Tips on Preventing Difficult Behavior

Whenever possible, preventing difficult behavior is better than trying to stop it once it has begun. Good observation skills are necessary to identify subtle changes in behavior early and to anticipate situations that are likely to create problems. Often the clues are nonverbal, such as an increase in restlessness.

Here are some suggestions for preventing difficult behavior from occurring:

- Simplify tasks, giving step-by-step instructions.

- Plan difficult tasks for times of day when fatigue is less.

- Reduce external confusion such as background noise or excess people or activity.

- Maintain a predictable routine to increase a sense of security and safety.

- Avoid too much idle time.

- Provide opportunities for positive experiences without overstimulation or unrealistic expectations.

- Speak in a calm, soothing tone of voice. Even when your words are no longer understood, the person with dementia may respond positively to the tone.

- Tailor activities to the level of functioning at the present, not what the person was able to do yesterday or even 1 hour ago.

- Be flexible enough to change plans.

- Avoid problem situations whenever possible.

- Monitor closely for medication reactions, illnesses, or injuries.

Coping with Difficult Behavior

When behavior problems occur despite your best efforts to prevent them, the first step is to try to determine the cause. If you can determine a reason for the behavior, the solution may become obvious. For example, if a bath is causing extreme agitation, postponing the bath may solve the problem.

Here are some general guidelines for handling behavior problems:

- Remain calm. Move slowly. Talk quietly. If you get upset, the behavior may get worse.

- Avoid arguing. These behaviors are neither rational nor deliberate so providing facts will not help and may only make the behavior worse.

- Ignore the behavior unless there is a safety risk. It may stop on its own.

- Divert the person to another activity such as going on a walk or listening to music, and the whole episode may be quickly forgotten.

- Remove the person from the situation or remove the cause of the behavior.

- Convey a sense of security and support.

- Respond to the underlying feelings that the behavior is expressing, such as fear or confusion.

- Use touch unless it might be interpreted as an attack.

- Leave and call for help if you are in any danger.

Other Sources of Help

Any abrupt change in behavior should be reported immediately to the doctor because it may indicate a delirium (see Chapter 3), an illness or injury that the person cannot describe, or a medication reaction (refer to Chapter 15).

If a persistent pattern of difficult behavior develops, keep a log describing the behavior itself, time of day, other outside events, and your responses; your doctor may be able to suggest other coping strategies. In some cases, medication can be helpful when all other approaches have failed (refer to Chapter 15).

Other sources of help include social workers or nurses who specialize in geriatrics or dementia, the local Alzheimer's Association, or support groups.

Repetitive Behavior

This group of behaviors includes repetitive questions and persistent demands or frequent telephone calls. It also includes repetitive motions, such as moving the tongue in and out.

Asking the same question repeatedly is a common early symptom of dementia and is often very irritating for families. It is usually either a direct result of short-term memory loss or an expression of anxiety, insecurity, or fear. It can also be caused by an inability to understand what is happening or difficulty communicating. It is not being done deliberately to annoy others, and it is not something the person with dementia can control.

The first step in coping with repetitive questions is to respond to the request, making sure that the answer is short and simple enough to be understood (refer to Chapter 12). Early in the illness it may work to write down the answer to a frequently asked question and put it in a central place, such as the kitchen table. Often questions concern the daily schedule. If a calendar showing a whole month is too complicated, listing a single day's activities may reduce anxiety about what is happening next. This approach will cease to be effective when the person with Alzheimer's disease can no longer read.

Try to understand and respond to the underlying feelings behind the repetitive questions or telephone calls. Frequently it is a search for security in the midst of a strange and frightening world. For example, if the person with dementia repeatedly asks when the Social Security check is coming, the real concern may be that there will not be enough money in the future. Reassurance that you are taking care of it and that there are ample funds may help reduce the fear and may be more effective than continuing to say that the Social Security checks always arrive on the third of the month. Similarly, giving a hug may do more than words to calm someone who is following you everywhere because of fear you will vanish.

Other coping strategies include:

- Discussing repetitive motions with the doctor. Sometimes they are a sign of problems with medications.

- Ignoring the behavior after the first response.

- Diverting the focus to another topic or activity.

- Providing increased structure to reduce anxiety. Someone

living alone and making frequent telephone calls may need a more protected living situation, such as a residential facility (see Chapter 17).

• Avoiding an argument.

Losing and Hiding Things

This behavior is common in dementia and is usually a direct consequence of either forgetfulness or suspicion. Prevention strategies include making sure that any valuable items are in a safe place. For example, Social Security checks should either go directly into the bank account or to the person managing the finances. Maintaining a predictable daily routine also helps keep things from being misplaced. For example, always putting dentures in a certain place at bedtime may reduce the number of times they cannot be found in the morning. Reduction of clutter in the home may also help prevent things from getting lost and/or make them easier to find.

When things do get lost, keep calm and provide reassurance. Arguing or asking where the item is will not help.

Withdrawal and Apathy

If you notice either withdrawal or apathy, ask yourself if there are any obvious reasons such as:

• Vision and/or hearing loss.

• Boredom.

- Communication problems.

- Depression (refer to Chapter 10).

- Reaction to a medication (see Chapter 15).

Withdrawal can be an appropriate response to overstimulation. If, however, you suspect that it is caused by boredom, see what happens if activities are increased.

Stubbornness

Stubbornness is a fairly common behavior in persons with Alzheimer's disease. It can interfere with important tasks and frustrate families who are trying to provide the best possible care.

It helps to understand why stubborn behavior occurs. It can sometimes be a result of anxiety or fear. Bathing, for example, can be a frightening experience for persons with dementia. Stubborn behavior can also be the result of fatigue, of short-term memory loss, of misunderstanding complicated directions, or being asked to do things that are no longer possible. It can also be a desperate attempt to maintain some control over a life that is slowly slipping away.

When you encounter stubborn behavior, remind yourself first that this is a result of the illness and is not being done deliberately to frustrate you. Then consider whether any of the following suggestions might help in your situation:

- Avoid rushing.

- Develop a predictable daily routine so tasks do not come as a surprise.

- Provide step-by-step instructions.

- Plan difficult tasks for the best time of day whenever possible.

- Modify expectations. For example, a full bath once a week with sponge baths in between may be sufficient.

- Reduce the number of decisions. Instead of asking whether the person is ready to take a bath, calmly announce that it is bath time.

- Delay the activity that is being resisted until later.

- Provide verbal and nonverbal reassurance to calm anxiety or reduce fear.

Consider hiring help for tasks such as bathing. Sometimes there is less resistance to the assistance of strangers than to family caregivers (see Chapter 16). If it is a new service that is being resisted, stick to the trial period described in Chapter 16.

Sleep Disturbances

Sleep problems are common with Alzheimer's disease and other dementing illnesses. Because lack of sleep may make behavior problems worse and also may interfere with the caregiver's rest, it is important to try to improve sleep patterns whenever possible.

Older persons in general require less sleep than younger ones. They also have more problems with insomnia than younger persons, and they frequently use sleeping medications (prescription and over-the-counter) to help them sleep better. Persons with Alzheimer's disease may already have experienced some sleep difficulties before the diagnosis of dementia was made, and the dementia may worsen the already existing sleeping problems. Sleeping medication should be avoided or used cautiously and only with the knowledge of the physician, because it may increase confusion, disorientation, or risk of falling caused by the dementia.

The first step in assessing sleep disturbances is to determine what is normal for that person in terms of amount of sleep required and usual bedtime. Then consider possible causes of sleep difficulties such as:

- Physical reasons, such as the pain of arthritis or the need to urinate.

- Too many daytime naps.

- Too little exercise.

- Too much alcohol or caffeine (coffee, tea, cocoa, or soft drinks).

- Irregular bedtime.

- Distractions in the sleeping area (too much noise or light).

- Depression (see Chapter 10).

- Side effects of medications (see Chapter 15).

Discuss and evaluate medication side-effects with the doctor. Maintain a regular bedtime schedule. Try increasing the amount of daily exercise or decreasing caffeine intake and, at the end of several weeks, evaluate whether there is any improvement in sleep.

Because caregiver exhaustion caused by sleep deprivation is a common reason for nursing home placement, it is potentially a serious problem when the caregiver is unable to get sufficient sleep. Before exhaustion occurs, explore ways of getting relief, such as enlisting the help of other people in the family or hiring a nighttime aide.

Sundowning

"Sundowning" is a term that describes increased restlessness and confusion occurring in the late afternoon, evening, or night. It is common in persons with dementing illnesses. The cause of sundowning is not understood, but it may have to do with factors such as increased fatigue at the end of the day or misinterpretation of cues in the immediate surroundings as darkness approaches. Some persons with Alzheimer's disease even reverse their days and nights. Sundowning can include wandering behavior (described in the next section).

If sundowning occurs, keep a careful log and discuss it with the doctor. There may be a treatable cause such as a delirium (see Chapter 3) or an infection (refer to Chapter 15). If possible, reduce the level of noise, activity, and demands on the person with Alzheimer disease at the end of the day. Medications are an option as a last resort (see Chapter 15).

Wandering

"Wandering" is a term used to describe either aimless or purposeful walking around. Although it is not present in all persons with dementing illnesses, it is fairly common and can lead to other serious problems, such as getting lost (described in Chapter 9). In its extreme form it can include agitated pacing. Sometimes the person who wanders is clearly looking for something (such as the bathroom) or someone ("my mother"). Other wanderers seem to have no goal in mind.

The Dangers of Wandering

Wandering can be dangerous. If the person with Alzheimer's disease wanders about the house at night without supervision, there may be safety hazards that need to be removed (refer to Chapter 9). If the person wanders outside, pedestrian accidents, exposure to extreme weather conditions, and mugging are all risks. Wandering in any location increases the chance of falling (described in Chapter 9).

Wanderers Require Constant Supervision

Wandering is a major stress on caregivers because persons who wander are often unpredictable and need constant watching. Wandering also forces families to deal with the balance between the need for safety and independence. Wandering can cause other services, such as an adult day care center, to refuse care. Although many persons who wander require institutional care because of the need for 24-hour supervision, some nursing homes refuse to admit wanderers. Sometimes the only option is a locked Alzheimer's unit either in a nursing home or a long-term psychiatric hospital (refer to Chapter 18). In some instances, admission to such facilities requires legal action (described in Chapter 14).

Explore Causes for Wandering

To look at possible causes for wandering, keep a log that includes the time of day, direction wandered, mood changes, trigger events, diet, and medications. Wandering can be a result of factors such as:

- Too much stimulation.

- Need for exercise.

- Fear or anxiety.

- Disorientation.

- Boredom.

- Delusions or hallucinations.

- Fear of upsetting tasks such as bathing.

- Previous work schedule.

- Need to use the toilet.

- Hunger.

Wandering can also be the result of medication side-effects, response to pain, acute illness, or dehydration. Recent location changes, such as a move or traveling, frequently lead to wandering as the person with dementia searches for home.

Prevention of Wandering

Consult your doctor if the wandering seems to be connected to medication, illness, injury, depression, hallucinations or delusions, or if it begins suddenly. Be sure your doctor knows about all medications, including over-the-counter ones. Modify the home so that wandering will be safe (see Chapter 9).

Think about using signs or pictures to show the way to the bathroom or disguising the door leading outside with a piece of cloth or a big poster. Install child-proof door knobs, special locks, or a bell on the door leading outside. Intercom systems or baby monitors enable you to hear into another room at night. Good lighting, including a nightlight, may be helpful. Consider enclosing the outside yard.

A schedule change may help. Reduce fluids after dinner and/or eliminate caffeine. Increase daytime activities and omit naps. Try going on walks together to satisfy the person's desire to be outside. Take the person to the bathroom every 2 hours during the day.

Other strategies include distraction, involvement in household chores, orientation to place, reassurance, or hiding shoes or coats to keep the person from wandering outside the home. Prevention of catastrophic reactions (described in the next section) that may lead to flight is also important.

What to Do When Wandering Occurs

If you think the person with Alzheimer's disease is about to wander, try diversion into other activities. Prevent nighttime wandering by providing reassurance and some orientation ("you are here in your bedroom and I am with you"). If nighttime wandering is common and interfering with your sleep, consider hiring an aide or asking other family members to help. Use of medications or restraints (such as a cloth vest restraint or a reclining chair with an attached tray) must be discussed with your doctor.

Make sure the person with Alzheimer's disease has identification on when going out. You can order a "Medic Alert" bracelet or necklace or have an ID engraved at a local jewelry store (refer to Chapter 9).

Agitated and Aggressive Behavior

While aggressive behavior including verbal or physical attacks and "catastrophic reactions" are not an inevitable part of dementia, people who are confused are more likely to become agitated. If this type of behavior does occur, it is usually in the middle stage of the illness when judgment is limited, frustration levels are high, and physical strength is still good. As with other behavior described in this chapter, it is important to see aggression as a symptom of the illness over which the person with Alzheimer's disease has no control. Beneath the aggression, the person is often fearful, anxious, frustrated, or lonely. Aggression is sometimes a defense against a perceived threat. For example, a new aide may be seen as an intruder coming into the home to steal something.

Families are often extremely shocked by any violent behavior in someone who has always been mild and kind, and when this aggression is directed toward caregivers, it becomes even more upsetting. Keep in mind that this is not a personal attack.

Catastrophic Reactions

A "catastrophic reaction" is an extreme response to stress by a person who has a dementia. It is often a symptom of overload when coping abilities have been stressed to the limit and some small incident becomes the last straw. Catastrophic reactions are most likely to happen when the person with dementia is fatigued, anxious, overstimulated, or faced with too many demands. Persons in the midst of a catastrophic reaction may be agitated, angry, anxious, tearful, stubborn, and extremely suspicious. They may pace, yell, or strike out. They are unable to control themselves.

Reasons for Aggressive Behavior

A careful assessment of aggressive behavior may identify a pattern. Look for a trigger event such as fatigue or a change in schedule; impaired vision or hearing that lead to misinterpretation; symptoms of pain; delirium (see Chapter 3); reactions to medications (see Chapter 15); or depression (see Chapter 10). Keep a log and call your doctor at once to discuss your observations. Sometimes medications or even hospitalization are indicated.

Coping with Aggressive Behavior

Although not always possible, prevention of aggression is a much better solution than trying to cope with it once it has begun. If there are situations that often lead to violent reactions, try to avoid them. Simplify the home (see Chapter 9) and maintain a predictable routine. Sometimes it is possible to identify the warning signs of agitation and interrupt them before they are out of control. Remove the person from the stressful situation or stop an activity that is upsetting. Keep calm yourself. Use nonverbal reassurance (touching) if you think it will not provoke an attack.

If violent behavior occurs, get help immediately. Do not tolerate any physical abuse. If the person is a danger to self or others, an involuntary admission to a psychiatric unit for several days of observation is usually possible. Call the police, local hospital emergency room, or your doctor to initiate the process. Restraints should be used only when ordered by the doctor and for a limited time under close supervision.

Antisocial Behavior

Socially inappropriate behavior and illegal activity such as shoplifting are uncommon, but if they do occur they are extremely embarrassing and upsetting to families. They are, however, a result of brain damage that leads to loss of control and loss of the sense of what behavior is appropriate. The main risk of this type of behavior is that it may cause families to isolate themselves further to avoid another embarrassment.

Socially inappropriate behavior can include such things as undressing in public, forgetting to dress, or urinating in unacceptable places. This behavior is often misinterpreted as sexual when it is actually a symptom of short-term memory loss, poor judgment, or confusion.

Socially inappropriate behavior can also include sexual behavior such as masturbation in public, sexual remarks or advances to strangers, or accusations regarding the spouse's fidelity. This behavior is a consequence of the loss of social inhibition, disorientation (mistaking the home care aide for the spouse), or improper interpretation of what is happening around them.

Coping with Antisocial Behavior

Overreacting or confronting the person with dementia will make matters worse. Remove the person from the situation or divert attention elsewhere. Explain to others that this behavior is a symptom of the illness, not a deliberate action. Consult the doctor if the behavior persists or if it begins to interfere with needed care.

Look for reasons behind such behavior. Is the person disrobing because of a need to use the toilet, because it is too warm, or because the person is fatigued and wants to go to bed? Is the behavior a consequence of boredom? If the person thinks the wastebasket is actually a toilet, is there a way to provide cues to help locate the bathroom? If the person repeatedly undresses, is it possible to modify the clothing to make it less easy to take off?

Hallucinations and Delusions

"Hallucinations" refer to seeing or hearing things that are not there whereas "delusions" are beliefs not founded in reality. Either may be a part of the disease itself or a result of other factors such as a reaction to a medication (see Chapter 15), a delirium (refer to Chapter 3), an infection, problems hearing, or improper lightening. Notify your doctor if you suspect any medical causes. If the hallucinations or delusions become disruptive, small doses of medication are sometimes helpful (see Chapter 15).

Arguing or confronting will not help. Instead, try to view these behaviors as a result of the loss of ability to interpret the external world; of anxiety or insecurity; or of disorientation to person, place, or time. It is common for persons with Alzheimer's disease to be convinced that their parents are still living. Remember that for them childhood may be the only part of their memory that is left, and their mother may represent one remaining piece of security in the midst of total confusion. Ignore harmless hallucinations and delusions and provide reassurance, diversion, and support.

Summary

Coping with all the change in functioning, emotions, and behavior is a major challenge for families. Part of the strategy for dealing with change is learning how to communicate with someone who has a dementing illness. Communication is the topic of the next chapter.

Chapter 12

Communication

The topic of this chapter is communication with persons who have Alzheimer's disease. How the illness affects communication, general communication tips, and communication challenges at each stage of the illness are summarized. Because communication is a complex topic and because maintaining communication is a key to providing good care, readers are strongly encouraged to obtain a copy of the book *Coping with Communication Challenges in Alzheimer's Disease* in the same *Coping with Aging Series.*

How Alzheimer's Disease Affects Communication

Communication, an important brain activity, is gradually lost as Alzheimer's disease progresses. This includes the ability to both send and receive information. It also includes verbal and nonverbal skills as well as ability to read.

Indeed, communication problems such as forgetting names or words are often early clues that something is wrong. Difficulty communicating is usually frustrating for both the person with Alzheimer's disease and others. Keep in mind that communication problems are not something the person with Alzheimer's disease can control.

General Communication Tips

Here are some ideas for effective communication with someone who has a dementing illness:

- Assess possible vision or hearing problems by arranging for a thorough eye and ear examination.

- Reduce background distractions, such as noise, confusion, and too many people, to increase concentration.

- Address the person by name.

- Speak slowly and clearly but not loudly, unless a hearing loss is present.

- Use simple words and short sentences.

- Maintain eye contact when talking or listening.

- Ask one question at a time.

- Allow time for a response.

- Avoid interrupting.

- Show interest. Be encouraging.

- Address the person as an adult.

- Offer only one idea or suggestion at a time.

- Discuss concrete events instead of abstract ideas.

- Ask direct "yes" or "no" questions instead of open-ended questions. Example: "Would you like to go for a walk?" instead of "What would you like to do now?"

- Help with word-finding if the person is becoming frustrated or anxious.

- Give one-step-at-a-time instructions.

- When repeating a statement, use the same words.

- Avoid correcting mistakes or arguing, quizzing the person, or giving orders. Be matter-of-fact and pleasant.

- Try again later if the person is fatigued or frustrated.

- Avoid announcing events too far in advance if you anticipate increased anxiety.

- Accept that "uncooperative" behavior may be a result of not understanding directions.

- Avoid talking about the person when the person is present.

- Side-step some questions. Example: If the person asks where mother is, ask about memories of mother rather than insisting she is no longer alive.

- Do not try to fill all the silences with talk. Sometimes just being together is enough.

The Importance of Nonverbal Communication

As the ability to communicate verbally is gradually lost, nonverbal communication becomes increasingly important. Reassuring gestures, calm tone of voice, touch, and smiles can all help convey what you are trying to say. Likewise, nonverbal communication by the person with Alzheimer's disease may help you fill in the verbal communication gaps. Often the underlying feelings are evident despite lack of meaning of what is said. Respond to underlying feelings, such as anxiety, by offering reassurance.

Communication at Each Stage

As with all behavior affected by Alzheimer's disease, the ability to communicate is often uneven. For example, the person may do well communicating face-to-face but not be able to comprehend what is said on the telephone. The ability to read words may be maintained while the meaning is lost.

The following is a brief description of major communication issues at each stage. For further information on the stages of Alzheimer's disease, refer to Chapter 5.

Early Stage

Communication problems often begin in subtle ways with word-finding difficulty or inability to follow conversations. Often the person with Alzheimer's disease recognizes these problems and feels frustrated along with others. Memory aides sometimes help at this stage. Continued stimulation is important as long as it is not overwhelming. This is the time to encourage the person to express feelings about the illness because the ability to do so will be lost later. If this occurs, others need to be good listeners and provide emotional support.

Middle Stage

Communication problems are much more obvious in this stage, and stress may make them worse. Withdrawal from social situations may occur as comprehension and interpersonal skills decline. Social interaction should be encouraged despite these difficulties in order to maintain communication abilities. Arrange for shorter visits or smaller groups. Reminiscing is a good strategy for encouraging conversation.

Late Stage

In this stage, the person with Alzheimer's disease is often unable to communicate needs or comprehend what others say. Nonverbal communication assumes greater importance. Others must now take their cues from key words or body language when assessing what the person wants or whether anything is wrong.

Summary

Communication is an essential part of maintaining a relationship with the person with Alzheimer's disease and providing good care. It is a topic beyond the scope of one chapter, therefore, readers are again encouraged to read the book *Coping with Communication Challenges in Alzheimer's Disease* in this *Coping with Aging Series.* The next chapter discusses how Alzheimer's disease changes families and how families learn to cope with the many challenges posed by this illness.

Chapter 13

Families: Finding Ways to Cope

The vast majority of people with Alzheimer's disease are cared for by their families. This chapter focuses on the challenges faced by those who care for relatives with dementing illnesses. It describes the impact of the illness on the family unit as well as on individual relationships within the family. Specific suggestions for recognizing and coping with the stress of caregiving are discussed. Finally, intervention and decisions about moving the person in with other relatives are addressed.

Impact on the Family

Caring for someone with Alzheimer's disease is an incredibly difficult and challenging task. Alzheimer's disease differs from most other illnesses because of its length, type of care required, and emotional stress on the people providing care ("caregivers").

Unlike an acute illness where families respond to a short-term crisis, Alzheimer's disease lasts many years and requires that families pace their involvement to avoid becoming totally exhausted. Unlike other illnesses that require primarily physical care, the care of someone with Alzheimer's disease involves managing complex issues such as behavioral change, safety, and restriction of independence. Unlike other illnesses that cause physical deterioration, families watch the person with Alzheimer's disease gradually lose the ability to think while still functioning physically. Furthermore, persons with Alzheimer's disease often look so healthy others may be less sympathetic with the stress the family is experiencing. And finally, the course of Alzheimer's disease is uncertain, calling for continual assessment and adaptation as the illness progresses.

Despite lack of choice about this unexpected responsibility, most families are tremendously dedicated to providing care and make up for their lack of experience with on-the-job training. They take pride in their work and frequently become so involved in providing care that they neglect their own needs.

Changes in Society Affect Family Caregiving

Families have changed significantly in the last 100 years. People live longer, have fewer children, and live longer distances apart. Providing care to elderly relatives has become more difficult as illustrated below:

- Spouses who provide care are older and often have their own health problems.

- Adult children who are caregivers are also older; many are already retired or in poor health themselves.

- Families are more spread out geographically. Adult children may live at a distance from their parents or the parents themselves may have retired to a different area.

- More women are employed, leaving less time and energy for caregiving.

- Divorce and remarriage of both the older and younger generation have complicated family relationships and affected caregiving.

Women are twice as likely as men to have the major responsibility of caring for someone with Alzheimer's disease. Spouses (usually older women) are the most common caregivers, followed by daughters, and then daughters-in-law. However, many caregivers are male spouses, many of whom are at least 75 years old.

Families Changed by Illness

Alzheimer's disease affects the whole family. It usually changes family patterns and relationships. It decreases leisure time and may affect responsibilities such as employment and parenting. It often alters communication among family members, disrupts normal routines, and changes expectations for the future. It may create financial stress. It frequently results in physical and emotional exhaustion.

Each member of the family, including the person with Alzheimer's disease, reacts in an individual way to the diagnosis. Common responses include: denial, shock, anger, sadness, anxiety, frustration, resentment, fear, helplessness, guilt, and depression. Each family member may respond differently to the illness, and this often leads to stress and conflict about issues such as the following:

Acceptance of the diagnosis. Often one or more family members continue to deny or minimize the illness longer than others.

Appropriate care at each stage. For example, it is common for some family members to stress safety whereas others feel strongly that independence should be preserved regardless of risks.

Sharing of caregiving responsibilities. If some in the family are overly involved in care and others are withdrawn, resentment, anger, and accusations of unfairness may result.

Adequacy of care. This includes care provided by family caregivers as well as community agencies.

One of the best ways to prevent or cope with family conflict is to involve a professional knowledgeable about Alzheimer's disease to provide information about the illness and its consequences, identify safety concerns, help develop a plan, offer support to caregivers and others in the family, and answer questions.

Other suggestions for reducing family conflict include:

- Allowing the relative who is slower in accepting the illness time to adapt.

- Arranging for periodic family meetings or telephone conference calls to share information, feelings, plans, and responsibilities.

- Attending caregiver support groups to learn more about the illness and get ideas from others.

- Obtaining and circulating medical reports and/or other information about Alzheimer's disease.

- Inviting the relative who is not accepting the illness or the need for care to visit the person for several days to see the situation first hand.

Family History Affects Caregiving

As the previous section describes, even for close-knit families, caring for someone with a dementing illness is a challenge. The stress of caregiving may be overwhelming for families who have had a history of other problems such as those listed below:

- Alcohol or drug abuse.

- Sexual abuse.

- Psychiatric illness.

- Unhappy marriage.

- Other family members needing special care.

- History of conflicts in relationships.

- Unemployment or financial stress.

It is impossible to pretend that family problems never occurred, and it may be unrealistic to fully repair a poor relationship. Anger, resentment, or escape into drug or alcohol abuse are common reactions when people feel pressured to become caregivers in such situations. With this history, it may not be a good idea to take on the full or even partial responsibility for the care of someone with Alzheimer's disease. Getting outside help and emotional support and setting definite limits are especially important.

Elder Abuse or Neglect

A small but growing number of the nation's elderly are victims of elder abuse or neglect that can include: physical harm, psychological trauma, lack of appropriate care, and financial exploitation. Most of these victims are abused or neglected by persons with whom they live and on whom they are dependent for care (usually relatives). Abuse and neglect occurs most often in families with a history of problems as described previously.

Persons with Alzheimer's disease and other dementing illnesses are especially vulnerable to abuse or neglect because of their confusion, lack of judgment, and inability to care for themselves. The stress of caring for someone with dementia can also lead to such frustration, resentment, and exhaustion that even the most well-intentioned relative loses control.

Symptoms of Abuse or Neglect

Clues that physical abuse or neglect may be occurring include: frequent injuries (burns, falls, bruises), malnutrition, dehydration, poor hygiene, refusal to allow outside help, and frequent hospital admissions. Warning signals of financial abuse include: transfer of assets or titles, significant changes in the life style of the caregiver or another person, missing items of value, unusual activity in bank accounts, misuse of credit cards, premature depletion of savings, and execution of a power of attorney or will when the person with Alzheimer's disease can no longer understand the document being signed. Because of the illness, it is unlikely that a reliable history of neglect or abuse can be obtained from the person with dementia.

Coping with Abuse or Neglect

If you suspect elder abuse or neglect, there are a number of approaches to take:

- Try to reach out to the caregiver by arranging for additional care if you think the problem is the result of caregiver limits or burnout. Encourage participation in a support group.

- Enlist the help of your doctor, social worker, nurse, or the local Alzheimer's Association.

- Discuss a change in living situation for the person with Alzheimer's disease and/or the caregiver. Perhaps it is time to relocate to a residential facility (see Chapter 17) or a nursing home (see Chapter 18) to obtain the needed care.

- Explore the state laws concerning elder abuse and neglect. States vary as to reporting requirements, confidentiality of reports, and allowed interventions.

- If the person with dementia is no longer competent to make decisions, talk to a lawyer about a court-appointed guardian. If the suspected abuser is already the guardian, explore the possibility of appointing someone else (refer to Chapter 14).

Impact on Marriage

When one partner in a marriage has Alzheimer's disease, the relationship is affected. This does not mean that it suddenly ceases to be satisfying, but it does mean that certain elements in the marriage will gradually change. Often before the diagnosis is made, the spouse consciously or unconsciously begins to compensate for the things the person with dementia can no longer do. How the marriage is affected depends on many factors such as the care required, personalities of each partner, and the history of the relationship. For example, people who have been married only a short time before the illness began will probably react differently than those who have been married many years.

Changes brought about by the illness often include the following:

- The necessity to take on new and unfamiliar roles. For example, a woman may have to learn to balance a checkbook for the first time or a male caregiver may have to learn to cook.

- Changes in routines.

- Loss of companionship, including physical and emotional support.

- Increased social isolation.

- Financial worries.

- Loss of future plans.

Spouses are faced with the sometimes overwhelming task of learning new skills, serving as an advocate, coordinating care, planning for the future, and making complex decisions alone. In addition, each stage of the illness poses new challenges.

Spouse caregivers (especially older women) are often unwilling to accept outside help. They frequently neglect their own health and become secondary casualties of the illness. They are at high risk of depression (described in Chapter 10).

Sexual Relationship is Affected

Regardless of age, the sexual relationship is an important part of most marriages and may change as a result of the illness. Sometimes persons with Alzheimer's disease lose interest in sex or are unable to recognize or respond to their partner's feelings. The caregiving spouse too may have little energy left to engage in sex and/or may no longer feel close because of changes in the relationship.

Other factors besides the dementia may explain changes in sexual interest or function such as medication side-effects, depression, or illnesses such as diabetes. Although it is difficult for most people to discuss such a personal matter with anyone else, doctors can help determine if these changes are caused by a treatable medical problem. You can also ask for a referral to a counselor skilled in this area. Many couples continue to feel physically close by holding and caressing one another, which is important since all human beings, including those with a dementing illness, need to feel loved.

On the other hand, sometimes persons with Alzheimer's disease show a greater interest in sex and may be overly aggressive. Later in the illness, the person with dementia may no longer recognize the spouse or may mistake others for the spouse, leading either to rejection or to inappropriate advances. Accusation of affairs is possible if the person with Alzheimer's disease becomes extremely suspicious. Moving to separate bedrooms is sometimes a solution. Sexual abuse should not be tolerated even if it is a symptom of illness.

Other Relationships or Divorce

The need for love and companionship continues throughout life. Marriage to someone with Alzheimer's disease, particularly in the later stages of the illness, may bring little or no satisfaction. If the person with Alzheimer's disease ceases to recognize the spouse, it may be devastating to the spouse. Spouses of persons with dementia may be in limbo for years. They are legally married to someone who has become a stranger, yet they cannot mourn the death because their spouse is still physically alive. In such circumstances, it is not unusual to think about forming a new relationship. This is an individual decision, having to do with religious and ethical beliefs, the history of the marriage, and the response of others, especially family. Talking to clergy or another professional might be helpful.

Some spouses consider divorce because the relationship has never been a happy one, because of changes in the relationship as a result of the illness, or because of legal or financial concerns (refer to Chapter 14). Especially in the latter case, it does not mean that the spouse has stopped caring about the person who is ill.

Impact on Adult Children

Adult children, especially daughters and daughters-in-law, provide a substantial amount of the care of people with dementing illnesses. They are often referred to as the "sandwich generation" because they are caught between the needs of their elderly relatives and their own families, careers, and leisure activities.

Adult children may have responsibility for all the care (known as "primary caregivers") or they may assist with the care provided by the spouse or someone else ("secondary caregivers"). They may live in the same household, across the street, or in another country. They may be 70 years old or young adults. They may always have had a close relationship with the parent or they may be estranged. Although some withdraw from taking on the caregiving role, most do what they can to help. They are, however, more likely to arrange for extra assistance from community agencies.

One issue that is common among adult children is concern about inheriting the same illness. Genetic testing is discussed in both Chapters 5 and 14.

Long-Distance Caregivers

Many adult children are geographically separated from the parent with dementia. If they have the sole responsibility for providing care, this is often stressful. Even if there is a spouse caregiver, adult children often worry about the toll the illness is taking on both parents. Guilt about being so far away and not doing more is common.

Recognizing the busy lives of their children, many spouse caregivers minimize their problems to avoid being a "burden." Unfortunately, this may eliminate an important source of emotional support and assistance that the children would want to provide. For adult children it may mean that they either continue to minimize the problems because of lack of accurate information, or they may worry even more because they suspect they are not being told the truth. Furthermore, protecting adult children from reality often backfires in a crisis when it is the children who have to come to the rescue and have no idea where to begin.

Long-distance caregivers need to find ways, such as the following, to monitor the situation and be prepared to step forward in a crisis:

- Identify important people in your relative's life, such as friends, neighbors, or clergy. Ask them to call you if they notice significant changes. Visit them when you are there.

- Know where important documents such as financial records, insurance papers, or durable power of attorney forms are kept.

- Know who the doctor is. Make sure the doctor knows how to reach you in an emergency.

- Develop an emergency plan for the care of the person with Alzheimer's disease should something happen to the primary caregiver (refer to Chapter 9).

- Even if the person with dementia does not yet need assistance from a community agency, explore what is available so you will be prepared in a crisis (see Chapter 16).

- If community agencies are involved, keep in touch by phone or letter and arrange meetings when you visit.

- Consider hiring a case manager to evaluate needs and arrange and monitor services (refer to Chapter 16).

Impact on Young Children

As part of the family, children of any age are also affected when a relative has Alzheimer's disease. The relative may be a parent or a grandparent and may live in the same household or far away. The children are affected both by their parents' worry and responsibilities for care as well as by the changes in their relationship with the person who has dementia.

The reactions of children to Alzheimer's disease vary greatly but may include:

- Fear that the disease is contagious and that they or their parents will "catch" it next.

- Guilt that something they did or thought caused the illness.

- Resentment that their parents are not as available to them.

- Anxiety or embarrassment about strange and unpre-dictable behavior and reluctance to invite friends home.

- Anger that they are having to take on adult responsibil-ities because others are busy providing care.

Because children are masters at sensing concerns of adults, trying to protect children from the stresses of the situation is impossible and often results in even worse fears than if the subject is discussed openly. Explanations need to be based on the child's age and ability to understand. There are some excellent books for children about Alzheimer's disease. Check your local library or the Alzheimer's Association. Consider asking the doctor, nurse, or social worker to talk to the child.

Watch for Behavior Problems

Children often express their distress through their behavior. Here are some signals that extra support or professional help may be needed:

- Nightmares or difficulty sleeping.

- Bed-wetting.

- Vague physical complaints.

- Withdrawal or depression.

- Problems in school.

- Antisocial behavior.

Talk to the teacher, school counselor, social worker, or the child's pediatrician.

Caregiver Stress

Stress is unavoidable when someone you love has Alzheimer's disease. The goal is to manage the stress so that it is not overwhelming.

Recognizing Caregiver Stress

In 1992 the National Institute of Mental Health estimated that 70 percent of caregivers experience stress that seriously affects their quality of life. It also estimated that as many as 15 to 30 percent of persons who care for disabled elderly relatives may have a depressive illness (refer to Chapter 10 for symptoms of depression). Both stress and depression develop so gradually that they are often not recognized until a crisis occurs.

Guilt is a common feeling among caregivers and increases caregiver stress. It often stems from normal feelings of anger and resentment at the relentless demands of providing 24-hour care. Guilt also occurs when caregivers have unrealistic expectations of themselves, such as never losing patience or when families wish for death to come.

Caregiver stress varies with the stage of the illness, amount and type of care required, nature of the relationship, living arrangement, financial resources, and age and health of the caregiver. What is stressful for one person may not be for another. No one, however, escapes stress altogether.

Here are some of the warning signals of caregiver stress:

- Chronic emotional and physical exhaustion.

- Irritability, frustration, anxiety, or anger.

- Health problems.

- Diminished involvement with friends and activities.

- Problems in relationships.

- Inability to perform as well at work.

- Worry about money.

- Low sense of self-esteem.

- Excessive guilt.

- Increased use of alcohol or drugs.

- Tearfulness.

- Refusal to allow anyone else to help.

- Feeling trapped.

These warning signals are clues that suggest that caregivers may need to find ways to alleviate some of their responsibility and stress.

Prevention of Caregiver Stress

All of the specific strategies for preventing caregiver stress can be summed up by saying that caregivers must take care of themselves. It is the only way to continue to provide care and to have the necessary patience to do a good job. It is not selfish for caregivers to think of their own needs. Indeed, if caregivers do not take care of themselves, they too are likely to become ill, often resulting in the person with dementia being placed outside the home.

The key to taking care of yourself as a caregiver is to recognize that no one can care for a person with Alzheimer's disease alone and that asking for help is not a sign of weakness. Prevention of caregiver stress is better than trying to deal with it after exhaustion sets in. Here are some specific suggestions for prevention of caregiver stress:

- At the time the diagnosis is made, think about ways to prevent caregiver stress from developing. Set aside specific times when you will get out of the house to do something enjoyable.

- Be good to yourself. Give yourself credit for a job well done instead of focusing on the times when you lose patience. Treat yourself to something special now and then to give yourself a lift: fresh flowers, a new book, a ticket to a baseball game, or a massage.

- Stay involved with friends, church or synagogue, and in activities you enjoy.

- Have fun. Go to a concert, movie, or dinner with friends. Go fishing or bowling. Work in your garden. Escape by reading a good book. Even a few minutes of fun or a good laugh each day will help.

- Get some exercise. Meet a friend for a walk several times a week or join an exercise program.

- Take care of your health. Get enough sleep, eat a well-balanced diet, see your doctor regularly, take your medications, and avoid over-use of alcohol or drugs.

- Set priorities and limits to simplify your life. You may not have enough energy or time to keep a spotless home or a perfect yard and prepare gourmet meals.

- Learn all you can about Alzheimer's disease and the resources in your community. Information helps you feel in control, have realistic expectations of the person in your care, and make appropriate future plans.

- Avoid thinking you are the only one who can provide adequate care. Although it is true that no one will do it exactly as you do, it is good for the person with Alzheimer's disease to see other people.

- Ask for help rather than waiting for others to volunteer. Most people want to help but need to be told what to do. Have a list handy of errands, things that need fixing, and times when you need to go out. A list of suggestions for things others can do to help is found in Chapter 16.

- Take a day at a time but make necessary plans for the future so you feel prepared.

- Share the tough decisions, such as limiting independence, with others. You need the support, and it will lessen any guilt feelings you may have later.

Once the person with Alzheimer's disease can no longer be left alone, all of these suggestions become harder to follow. Nevertheless, you need to plan regular breaks from caregiving each week. Enlist the help of family or friends or arrange for services from a community agency (described in Chapter 16). Not doing so may hasten the day when your relative must move to a residential facility or nursing home because you are exhausted or ill.

Monitoring Caregiver Stress

Because caregivers often do not recognize the extent to which they are stressed or even depressed, this needs to be monitored by family or others on a regular basis. In some instances it is necessary for caregivers to physically or emotionally withdraw to survive. If there is any sign that the caregiver is seriously depressed or suicidal, other relatives should contact the doctor immediately.

Some caregivers strongly resist outside help despite clear risks to their own health from the stress of singlehandedly providing care. Some of the reasons for reluctance to use community agencies are described in Chapter 16. If this happens, first try to determine what the reason is. For example, if it is financial, would the caregiver accept help if others in the family paid for the service? If the caregiver is overwhelmed at the thought of finding and arranging services, could someone else do this task?

If the primary caregiver's health is at risk, other family members should consider calling the physician or another professional and asking for help. If the caregiver is too ill to provide adequate care or has other problems such as alcohol abuse that threaten the health or safety of the person with dementia, it may be necessary to intervene legally (see Chapter 14).

Support Groups

Caregiver support groups are one way to help families learn about the illness and community resources, share feelings, and find new ideas for providing care and coping with stress. Often sponsored by the Alzheimer's Association, they are usually open to caregivers as well as other relatives. In large metropolitan areas, there may be special groups for specific people such as adult children, male caregivers, or even those diagnosed with early Alzheimer's disease. Support groups reduce the isolation commonly experienced by caregivers.

Support groups are not for everyone. Some people prefer to get the support they need from family, friends, clergy, or other organizations to which they have belonged for many years. Some people get information about the disease by reading. Others do not feel comfortable sharing feelings in a group. Some, when they have only limited time to get away, prefer to do something fun rather than think about Alzheimer's disease. What is important is that caregivers find ways to get needed support that work for them.

When and How to Intervene

One of the most complex issues facing families is determining how long to allow persons with Alzheimer's disease the dignity of making their own decisions before beginning to intervene. It raises ethical and sometimes legal questions and is often an agonizing decision for caregivers to make. Here are some factors to consider:

- Safety both for the person with Alzheimer's disease and others.

- Potential for exploitation.

- Danger to physical health from untreated medical conditions or self-neglect.

- Squandering financial resources needed for future care because of inability to manage money.

Moving in with Relatives

One option when someone with Alzheimer's disease needs more care or supervision is to move in with relatives. This is a major decision and requires careful thought and time to explore the pros and cons. Consider the following questions:

- Is the person with dementia still competent to make decisions? If so, how does the person feel about leaving friends and familiar surroundings and living with you?

- Can you provide the required care?

- Are there community services in your area to help?

- Is there room? Will there be enough privacy for everyone?

- If you have a spouse or children, how do they feel about this idea? Will your home be too noisy or busy for someone with Alzheimer's disease?

- If you are employed, who will care for the person when you are at work?

- What kind of relationship have you had with the person who has dementia?

Consider getting an outside opinion from a professional or arranging for an extended trial visit of several months before making a final decision.

No Right Answers

Individual members of a family frequently see the same situation very differently and often disagree about the course of action. Some people in the family, for example, may feel strongly that the person with Alzheimer's disease should remain independent in spite of obvious risks to safety, whereas others may feel equally strongly that safety is more important. Others may deny any problems at all. These differences often lead to conflict about what to do.

Unfortunately, there is no formula to resolve differences and arrive at an acceptable plan for every situation. Any decision that is made will carry its own risk. It is never possible to anticipate all the consequences of even the most well thought out plan. For example, if a family insists that a person with Alzheimer's disease move to a residential facility, safety risks may decrease at the same time that the risks of greater disorientation or even depression may increase.

Enlist Outside Help

A fresh look at your situation by an experienced professional may help both to objectively assess risks and decide whether, how, and when to intervene. Possible sources of help include the doctor, nurse, social worker, case manager, visiting nurse, or occupational therapist. Support groups almost always include family caregivers who have struggled with similar issues and whose solutions may be relevant.

Summary

Families are the unsung heroes in the care of persons with Alzheimer's disease. The main message of this chapter, however, is that no one can singlehandedly care for someone with a dementing illness. Another responsibility of families is to begin future planning as soon as the diagnosis is made. Legal and financial planning are discussed in the next chapter.

References

National Institute of Mental Health. (1992). Fact Sheet: *Mental Health and Aging: Older Women*.

Chapter 14

Financial and Legal Planning

Financial and legal planning are discussed in this chapter, including the need for advanced planning, getting financial and legal affairs in order, and the importance of involving family in these efforts. Specific financial programs and legal documents are reviewed and suggestions made for finding appropriate advisors.

The Importance of Financial and Legal Planning

Financial and legal planning are more important for Alzheimer's disease than for most other illnesses for the following reasons:

- The illness eventually renders the person with Alzheimer's disease incapable of managing financial, legal, and personal affairs.

- The illness lasts many years, is progressive, and requires increasingly expensive care that is usually not covered by private insurance or Medicare and can impoverish the spouse.

- In the terminal stage, families are often faced with complex decisions about prolonging life.

Start Planning Early

Ideally, financial and legal planning should begin at the time of the diagnosis. As suggested in Chapter 4, one of the questions to ask the physician at the time of diagnosis is whether the person with dementia is capable of making personal, legal, and financial decisions (is "legally competent"). The diagnosis of Alzheimer's disease does not usually mean that persons are suddenly unable to handle their own affairs. Indeed, one major reason for seeking an early evaluation and sharing the diagnosis with the person who has Alzheimer's disease is to involve the person in making future plans.

If the illness is diagnosed early, it is important to encourage as much independence as possible while at the same time planning for future incapacity. The role of caregivers, other relatives, or advisors will change as the illness progresses. Help with monitoring and organizing affairs may later be replaced with joint management. Eventually, however, someone else will have to assume total responsibility for all financial and legal matters. Legal and financial planning should be an ongoing process because laws may change during the course of the illness, requiring a different approach.

Goals of Financial and Legal Planning

The main goals of financial and legal planning are to:

- Manage funds to provide needed care.

- Protect the financial security of the spouse or dependent children.

- Assure a smooth transfer of responsibility when the person with Alzheimer's disease can no longer make financial, legal, medical, and other personal decisions.

Family Involvement

For most people, financial and legal matters are private. They often symbolize adulthood when one maintains independence and control over one's own life. Because caregivers or other relatives are often uncomfortable about intruding, the initial approach needs to be carefully and sensitively planned. One approach is for the family to use the diagnosis to call a meeting to begin necessary planning for the future. The focus should be on how to manage funds to provide care in the future, not on whether there will be an inheritance left. Expressing genuine concern and offering assistance rather than trying to take over may also reduce resistance or suspicion about motives. Difficult as this discussion may be, putting it off may mean that these issues will have to be dealt with in a crisis. Ask for help from someone else such as a clergy, bank officer, doctor, lawyer, or counselor if you need assistance in introducing this topic. It may be wise to ask one family member to prepare written minutes of meetings to reduce future misunderstandings or conflicts.

How Families Can Help

Some spouses (especially older women) may never have had responsibility for financial and legal affairs in their marriages. Although many rise to the challenge and master needed skills, others may be too exhausted or stressed by caregiving to even try. In such cases, other relatives, trusted friends, or paid advisors need to provide assistance. They can help in many ways including: paying bills, filling out insurance claims, preparing tax returns, exploring investment possibilities, and assisting with decision making. Adult children, although not legally responsible for their parents, can help pay for specific services. Even relatives living at a distance can assist with financial and legal tasks.

Recognize Caregiver Mortality

As discussed in Chapter 9, it is wise to have a back-up plan for care of the person with Alzheimer's disease if the caregiver becomes ill or dies. This applies as well to legal and financial affairs and is another reason to make sure that others in the family, in addition to the primary caregiver, are knowledgeable about this topic.

Getting Affairs in Order

Mismanagement of financial and legal affairs is often an early symptom of the illness. It is common to discover disconnection, eviction or overdraft notices, lapses in insurance policies, or problems with tax returns.

The first step in any financial or legal planning is to get current affairs in order. This may be easier said than done if the person with dementia has lost or hidden important documents and cannot find them. Sometimes a thorough search of the house is necessary. Look for the following records:

- Income sources and amounts, savings and investments, bank accounts, trust account statements, debts (including mortgages), credit cards, tax records (income and property), pension information, and stock certificates.

- Insurance policies (life, health, disability, property, automobile, and long-term care).

- Social Security number; military records; birth, marriage, and divorce certificates; citizenship papers; and safe deposit box key and list of contents.

- Contracts, deeds, leases, durable powers of attorney for health care and financial management, living wills, wills, codicils, and trust agreements.

- Burial and funeral arrangements.

- Names of advisors such as accountant, broker, financial planner, lawyer, and clergy.

Prepare a master list of the information and give copies to other family members and important advisors. The list should be periodically updated and distributed.

Make sure all records are in an appropriate place and that others know where to find them. For example, a durable power of attorney for health care should be kept in an obvious place, such as in a desk drawer or on a bulletin board, instead of in a safe deposit box.

Financial Planning

Once financial affairs are organized, determine whether resources are adequate to meet current needs and, if not, explore options either to reduce expenses or to increase income.

Determine which financial tasks the person with Alzheimer's disease can still do independently and which require assistance. If financial affairs are in good order, periodic monitoring may be all that is necessary at first. If, on the other hand, the financial affairs are in disarray, it may be necessary either to share all the day-to-day financial tasks or to take over completely.

Here are some suggestions for routine financial management:

- Review mail regularly.

- Arrange for direct deposit of checks into the bank.

- Explore special bank accounts that enable someone else to monitor spending (dual signature or power-of-attorney accounts are examples).

- Provide a small allowance so that the person with dementia has some independence. Do not let the person carry large sums of money.

- Investigate becoming a payee for Social Security. A physician's statement that the person with Alzheimer's disease is no longer capable of handling money is required.

- Withdraw large amounts from accessible accounts to reduce the possibility of exploitation or uncontrolled spending. Cancel credit cards if necessary.

- Redirect mail to the address of the person paying the bills.

- Avoid discussion of financial matters if the person with Alzheimer's disease becomes anxious or agitated. Provide reassurance that you are taking care of things.

Plan for the Future

The first step in planning for the future is to prepare a durable power of attorney for financial management, a document in which another person (usually a relative) is appointed to manage the financial affairs when the person with Alzheimer's disease is no longer able to do so. With such a durable power of attorney, guardianship or conservatorship proceedings can often be avoided. The person signing a durable power of attorney must be legally competent at the time the document is executed. Although some states have standard power of attorney forms, it is always wise to consult an attorney because the standard form may go either too far or not far enough in powers granted. There is a risk of financial abuse with a financial power of attorney because there is no court oversight or required accounting; however, a lawsuit for misuse of the power of attorney is sometimes possible.

Anticipate the need for more care as the illness progresses and begin exploring the costs of care in your community. Investigate whether insurance will pay for any care. Compare the costs of home care with the costs of residential facilities or nursing homes. Find out whether any financial assistance will be available. Keep in mind that it is often difficult to get into a nursing home on Medicaid without an initial period of private pay. Be sure to keep a log of all your telephone calls when you are doing this.

Enlist the Help of Experts

Consult an expert such as a banker, attorney, accountant, financial planner, or counselor to help with long-range financial planning. If you do not already have an advisor, call the senior center, Alzheimer's Association, or Bar Association nearest you. Senior centers or offices on aging sometimes have volunteers or paralegal staff to help with insurance paperwork or simple tax returns.

Financial Assistance Programs

As discussed in Chapter 16, there are few public or private funding sources to help pay the costs of care. The financial assistance that is available varies greatly from state to state in terms of eligibility, coverage, and agencies operating the programs.

Federally run programs are fairly consistent across the country. They include:

Social Security Retirement. Available at a reduced rate beginning at age 62 or at the full rate at age 65. Contact the Social Security Administration.

Supplemental Security Income (SSI). Run by the Social Security Administration, it provides income for those whose incomes and assets are below the poverty level.

Social Security Disability. Disability income for people who meet strict disability criteria and who are under age 65. Apply at the Social Security office. If the initial or subsequent applications are denied, be sure to file appeals.

Medicare. Helps pay for hospital and physician charges as well as some home health care, hospice care, and short-term skilled care in a nursing home. Because people with Alzheimer's disease often do not meet the medical criteria for Medicare funding, be sure to check first with the home health agency or nursing home.

Qualified Medicare Beneficiary Program (QMB). Provides assistance with Medicare premiums, deductibles, and co-insurance for persons with low incomes and assets. Contact the local social service or welfare department.

Veterans Administration Pensions. For veterans who are "service-connected" or low income. Contact the nearest Veterans Administration office.

Veterans Administration Health Care. Hospital and nursing home care available to certain categories of veterans. Call the nearest VA hospital.

Public programs that are funded by combinations of federal, state, or local dollars vary from state to state. The agencies responsible have different names such as: welfare, public assistance, social services, or human services. Many people have strong feelings about applying for welfare. It may help to remind them that these programs are supported by taxes that they have paid all their lives to help others in need. Programs to explore include:

Food Stamps. Helps people who are at the poverty level buy food.

Assistance with energy bills. Contact the utility company.

Medicaid (also known as Medical Assistance or Title 19). Pays for health care expenses, including care from doctors, hospitals, home health agencies, and nursing homes. Covered services vary greatly. Eligibility is based on limited income and assets. Transferring assets (divestment) is prohibited within 30 months of applying. Not all home care agencies, doctors, or nursing homes accept Medicaid payments. Co-payments are sometimes required. Because the Medicaid law is always changing and varies from state to state, legal advice is recommended. Refer to Chapter 18 for a discussion of Medicaid payment for nursing home care.

Other possible sources of financial help include tax programs such as property tax deferral, rent rebates, or claiming parents as dependents on income tax returns. Reverse mortgages or home equity conversions are allowed in some states and provide income for those who are "house rich" but "cash poor." Nonprofit community agencies may have sliding fee scales for services. Cashing in life insurance policies may be an option.

Private Insurance. Private health insurance coverage is extremely variable. For example, some health insurance will pay for home health or hospice care whereas others do not. Long-term care insurance policies are relatively new, so claims experience is limited. However, it is too late to take out a long-term care policy after the diagnosis of dementia is made. If you already have such a policy, do not assume it will pay for everything you need. Check to see if it includes home care or residential care. Is prior hospitalization required? Is the care in a nursing home restricted to a certain level? For example, many persons with Alzheimer's disease only require supervision (custodial care) whereas many insurance policies only reimburse if skilled nursing care is needed. Check with your state insurance commissioner's office if you have any problems with private health insurance policies.

Special Financial Issues

Retirement. If the person with Alzheimer's disease is employed, retirement because of disability will eventually be necessary. Discuss this with your physician first to make sure the illness is well documented. Find out whether there is any private disability policy. Apply for Social Security Disability; it usually takes 6 months until eligibility is determined.

Employed Caregivers. Think carefully about the pros and cons of giving up your job. How will you manage with this loss of income? Does getting out of the house to work help you cope with the pressures of caregiving? Are there community services that can care for your relative when you are at work? Is it possible to work part-time or at home, job share, or take a leave of absence? Discuss your situation with your employer. Some large companies have employee assistance programs that provide counseling or information about resources.

Uncontrolled Spending. The judgment of persons with Alzheimer's disease is affected by the illness and sometimes results in excessive spending. If this occurs, consider canceling bank accounts and credit cards. If you do not have the legal authority to do so, a guardian or conservator appointed by the court may be necessary to assure that funds needed for future care are not squandered.

Financial Abuse Or Neglect. Persons with Alzheimer's disease are vulnerable to financial exploitation. They may invite strangers into their homes, become victims of unscrupulous insurance agents or other scams, display large sums of money in public, pay for the same expensive item or service many times over, or purchase insurance or annuities that are unsound investments given their illnesses. They may also be pressured by relatives to divest their assets, thereby disqualifying them from receiving Medicaid in the future. Refer to Chapter 13 for a full discussion of financial abuse.

Genetic Testing. In families where there is a strong history of dementia, younger relatives sometimes request genetic testing for the inherited form of Alzheimer's disease described in Chapter 5. The risks of this step need to be explored with an attorney. Risks include possible future disqualification from medical or long-term care insurance.

Legal Planning

As described earlier in this chapter, locating and listing the existing legal documents is the first step in financial and legal planning.

Find a Legal Advisor

It is usually wise to have a legal advisor. This could be a family attorney or a lawyer specializing in "elder law." Call the local Bar Association or the Alzheimer's Association if you need suggestions or references. In some areas there are low-cost legal aid clinics, public interest law firms, or paralegal programs that provide assistance to the elderly. Be sure to ask about the advisor's experience. Many lawyers do not keep up with legal changes in the Medicaid program or handle guardianship or conservatorship matters. Ask about the cost of preparing legal documents or obtaining legal advice. Some attorneys have a flat fee for a specific task (such as preparing a power of attorney) whereas others bill by the hour.

When the Person is Competent

If the person with Alzheimer's disease is still legally competent (refer to the beginning of this chapter for a definition of legal competence) the following legal documents should be prepared or reviewed as soon as possible: durable power of attorney for finances (described earlier), a will, and an advance directive for health care.

A will consists of written instructions for how assets are to be handled after death. Wills should be reviewed every 5 years or if the marital status, state law, or state of residence has changed since it was signed.

An advance medical directive is a written document that specifies what kinds of medical care you would want if you were no longer able to speak for yourself. There are two main types of advance directives: a living will and a durable power of attorney for health care.

A living will provides instructions about medical care in the event of a terminal illness or a persistent vegetative state or an irreversible coma. It might include such topics as the use of breathing machines and feeding tubes.

Many states have standard forms for living wills that are usually available from your doctor or local hospital.

A durable power of attorney for health care gives advance opportunity to appoint someone (usually a relative) to make health care decisions in the event of incapacity. Specific instructions about medical care can be included. Many states have standard forms that your doctor or local hospital can provide. Even relatives now need to be gran-ted the legal right to make medical decisions for another adult.

Be sure your doctor and hospital have copies of the living will or power of attorney for the medical record and that the person with Alzheimer's disease has an ID card indicating who has been chosen to make medical decisions. Keep the original in an easy place to find at home. Some states have procedures for registering advance directives with a public agency. The organization Choice in Dying also has a registry service (see Chapter 19). Both the living will and the durable power of attorney for health care only go into effect if a health care professional (usually a doctor) certifies that the person is no longer able to understand the issues and make decisions.

Some states have passed laws permitting "surrogate" (substitute) decision makers for health care for people who do not have a living will or power of attorney for health care or whose written advance directives do not apply to the medical issues that arise.

Discuss Health Care Instructions Early

Advance directives for health care work best when families have discussed these issues ahead of time. While the person with Alzheimer's disease can still think clearly, it is important for family members to determine what he or she would want done if critically ill. A complete list of topics to discuss is found in Chapter 19.

Knowing what persons with Alzheimer's disease would want helps families make decisions that fit the persons' unique beliefs and values. It also minimizes the risk of conflict in the family and between the family and health care staff. It reduces the guilt that families often feel when they are forced to guess what the ill person would have wanted. Finally, with advance directives, guardianship of the person is often avoided.

If the person with Alzheimer's disease has already been named in someone else's power of attorney as the person who will be responsible for decisions, this should be changed.

Living Trust

In addition to the legal documents just described, an optional legal document is a living trust, which transfers assets into a trust managed by a trustee. This is usually only appropriate when large sums of money are involved or with more modest sums when there is no appropriate person for the durable power of attorney for financial management. A living trust needs to be prepared by a lawyer. It should be drafted so it does not interfere with future eligibility for Medicaid. Beware of do-it-yourself living trusts or high pressure sales people who try to "sell" trust agreements that are not tailored to the client's needs and wishes or to state law.

Incompetency

All persons with Alzheimer's disease eventually become incompetent and unable to manage their own affairs. Not all persons with dementia, however, need court-appointed guardians or conservators. Those who have signed powers of attorney for finances and health care while they were still competent often avoid guardianships.

Guardianship

"Guardianship" is a court proceeding initiated by family or other interested parties with the help of an attorney. Medical proof of incompetency is usually needed. Sometimes there must also be evidence of danger to self (such as malnutrition) or to others (such as fires). Guardianship is a time consuming, complicated, and often upsetting process that should be the last resort; however, it is sometimes unavoidable.

A guardian may be appointed only to manage money (guardian of estate or conservatorship) or only to make personal decisions (guardian of person) or both. Usually relatives are appointed as guardians or conservators and are required to report periodically to the court. Supervision of guardians by the court varies greatly. If a guardian is not acting in the best interests of the person with dementia, the court should be petitioned to appoint another.

Guardians are sometimes prohibited from actions such as admitting the person with dementia to a psychiatric hospital unless specific permission is granted by the court. In some situations, the court may order the person with Alzheimer's disease to be moved to a protected living situation such as a residential facility or a nursing home.

Special Legal Issues

Transferring assets. As mentioned earlier, divestment is prohibited within 30 months of applying for Medicaid. It is important to consult a qualified lawyer before disposing of any property to make sure that action does not result in future ineligibility for Medicaid. Remember that Medicaid law changes frequently.

Divorce. Some spouses of persons with Alzheimer's disease consider divorce because of changes in the relationship caused by the illness. Others consider it to avoid being impoverished by costs of care. Both the emotional and financial needs of the spouse are important and need to be carefully considered in any long-term financial and legal planning.

Summary

Planning ahead, obtaining information, and serving as an advocate are the keys to coping with the complex financial and legal issues that arise in the course of a dementing illness. Families also need to serve as advocates to ensure the person with Alzheimer's disease obtains regular medical care throughout the illness. Ongoing medical care is the subject of the next chapter.

Chapter **15**

Ongoing Medical Care

Persons with Alzheimer's disease require regular medical care throughout the course of their illness. In this chapter, suggestions for how to work with a number of health care professionals will be discussed. The symptoms of an acute illness or injury that may require medical attention are identified. Management of medications for persons with dementing illnesses is reviewed. Finally, what to expect when a person with Alzheimer's disease is hospitalized is described.

Working with Health Professionals

A number of different health care professionals can provide information and assistance to families caring for persons with dementia. Each of these professionals has a particular area of expertise and can be found in a variety of settings including hospitals, geriatric clinics, doctor's offices, home health care agencies, and community programs serving the elderly or disabled. Here are some of the professionals you are most likely to meet.

Physician

Finding a physician to provide regular medical care is important. It may not be the same physician who did the initial evaluation of the memory loss but needs to be someone who is experienced in caring for people with Alzheimer's disease, who is accessible, and who communicates well. Physicians who provide regular medical care to older adults are usually family practitioners or internists (refer to Chapter 4 for more information). The local

Medical Society or Alzheimer's Association can provide suggestions of skilled physicians. Schedule an appointment to describe your situation and to evaluate whether that doctor will be able to meet the needs of your relative.

Nurse

A nurse can help evaluate medical concerns, communicate questions to the doctor, and provide practical suggestions about caring for someone with Alzheimer's disease. You will not only get to know the nurse in your doctor's office but you may also need to use the services of a community nurse who will visit the home (refer to Chapter 16 for a description of home care services). Some nurses have advanced education in geriatrics and are certified as "geriatric nurse practitioners."

Social Worker

Social workers are responsible for helping families evaluate what community services may be helpful, make referrals, provide emotional support as the disease progresses, and help families work together. They can also offer suggestions for coping with communication problems or challenging behaviors.

Occupational Therapist

An occupational therapist can help evaluate safety, needs for special equipment, and appropriate everyday activities for the person with Alzheimer's disease. Occupational therapists work both in hospitals and home health agencies. A doctor's referral is needed to arrange for a home visit (see Chapter 16).

Physical Therapist

Physical therapists are responsible for evaluating and helping with mobility problems, including the risks and prevention of falls. They also work both in hospitals and home health agencies under the orders of a physician.

Other health care professionals who may be helpful are pharmacists, podiatrists, dietitians, speech pathologists, psychiatrists (refer to Chapters 4 and 10), and neuropsychologists (see Chapter 4).

The Role of the Family in Medical Care

Because persons with a dementing illness frequently cannot provide accurate descriptions of their health problems, families need to play a more active role in making sure they receive adequate medical care. Responsibilities include:

1. *Observing and reporting any significant changes.* For example, you need to be alert to symptoms described below that might signal a medical problem such as a urinary tract infection or a medication reaction.

2. *Providing recommended treatments.* This includes making sure medications are taken as scheduled and that adequate nutrition and hydration are maintained.

3. *Giving feedback about treatments.* For example, the doctor should be notified promptly if drowsiness or agitation occurs after starting a new medication.

4. *Serving as an advocate.* Because persons with Alzheimer's disease are unlikely to recognize changes and/or to take any initiative to obtain help, families need to be much more assertive than usual. Be sure the doctor has a copy of the durable power of attorney for health care or living will (see Chapter 14) and is willing to follow those instructions.

Communicating with Health Professionals

Here are some suggestions for communicating with your health care providers:

- Prepare for visits to the doctor by making a list of topics to discuss.

- Bring all the medications to doctor's appointments, including prescription and over-the-counter drugs.

- Describe symptoms in detail. Include: how long you have noticed this symptom, when it happens, how often it happens, and any pattern (such as a certain time of day or after taking a particular medication). Keeping a log may help you remember details.

- Ask questions if you do not understand explanations or instructions.

- Take notes and review them before you leave to make sure you understand all recommendations.

- Be sure you know whom to call during the night or weekend if a problem arises.

Private Communication with Health Care Providers

Many relatives are not comfortable speaking frankly in front of a person with dementia during a clinic visit. However, it is important that the doctor hear the concerns of families. Ways of communicating should be discussed directly with the physician and a plan agreed on that preserves your relative's independence and dignity at the same time that it provides the doctor with necessary and accurate information. There are various ways to make sure this happens. One is to call in advance of an appointment and talk to the doctor or another person, such as the nurse or social worker. Another is to write the doctor a note before the visit, or finally, you can request a private meeting with the physician either in conjunction with that visit or at another time.

Providing Feedback to Health Professionals

Often families are reluctant to voice any reservations about suggestions made by health care professionals, but remember that you as family are the experts about your particular situation. Feel free to let your health care providers know if a recommendation is unrealistic so that you can work together to find a better solution.

When to Seek Medical Attention

Routine Care

People with dementing illnesses need the same routine preventive medical care as other adults in their age group, such as regular physical exams, vaccinations, eye, dental, and hearing exams. They should also be seen every 6 months to monitor the progress of their dementia and to evaluate what care might be helpful at each stage of the illness. You will need to take responsibility for making these appointments and assuring that your family member keeps them.

Illnesses or Injuries

Persons with Alzheimer's disease can also suffer from other illnesses or injuries, but they will become progressively unable to accurately report symptoms. Furthermore, the normal symptoms of an illness seen in younger persons may be absent. For example, there may be no pain with a urinary tract infection. Learn to observe signs that something is wrong, such as the following:

- Abrupt changes in behavior, function, or personality.

- Confusion or hallucinations.

- Increase in restlessness or moaning.

- Falls.

- Fever (report any fever over 101° F to your doctor).

- Vomiting.

- Diarrhea.

- Swelling of hands or feet.

- Difficulty breathing.

- Weight loss or gain.

- Pressure sores.

- Dehydration.

- Coughing.

- Constipation.

- Sudden change in ability to control urine.

- Refusal to eat or drink.

- Remaining in bed.

- Inability to walk.

- Extreme drowsiness.

- Seizures.

Trust your instincts. You know better than anyone else what is normal for this person. Do not assume that all changes are an inevitable progression of the illness and that nothing can be done. Any abrupt change from what is normal requires an evaluation.

Plan Ahead

Anticipating medical issues that may arise as the illness progresses is extremely important. Try to involve the person with Alzheimer's disease in these discussions if at all possible. A list of issues to think about is found in Chapter 19.

Medications

Any chemical, pill, drop, cream, potion, or lotion that in any way affects your body is a drug and should be considered a medication. Medications may be taken by mouth, inhaled, put on the skin, put into the eyes, inserted into the vagina, or taken as a rectal suppository. Medications include both those prescribed by your physician and over-the-counter medications. Alcohol, vitamins, dietary supplements, or other non-food products purchased in health food stores as well as caffeine contained in coffee, tea, chocolate, and cola drinks and nicotine contained in tobacco are drugs and should also be considered medications.

Because a common side effect of many medications in a person with Alzheimer's disease is worsening confusion, whenever possible it is best to avoid medications. Discuss alternatives to medications with the doctor. Never give the person with Alzheimer's disease any medication, including alcohol and caffeine, without the advice of the physician.

Take *All* Medications to the Doctor's Appointments

Whenever you take your family member to visit the doctor, it is a good practice to bring along all medications—both prescription and the over-the-counter. Be sure to let the doctor know the amount of alcohol, caffeine, and nicotine being consumed as well.

Reasons for Taking Medications

A person with Alzheimer's disease may take medication for three reasons:

- To help treat or prevent progression of dementia.

- To treat a medical problem unrelated to the dementia.

- To treat a problem that arises because of the dementia.

Medications to Treat or Prevent Progression of Dementia

As mentioned in Chapter 5, at the present time no medication exists to prevent or reverse the destruction of brain cells in Alzheimer's disease. If multi-infarct dementia is present, the dementia may improve or progression may be halted by controlling risk factors for stroke. This usually means keeping the blood pressure normal, taking one-half to one aspirin per day, and stopping smoking. If you have an irregular heart beat called "atrial fibrillation" you are more likely to have strokes than if you have a regular heart beat. It has been shown in large studies that strokes can be prevented in many persons with atrial fibrillation by regularly using blood thinners such as warfarin.

You or your family member may be asked to participate in a study that is investigating a medication for the treatment of Alzheimer's disease as discussed in Chapter 5. Be sure you understand the side effects that might occur from such a medication.

Medications to Treat Medical Problems Unrelated to the Dementia

As people grow older, they are increasingly susceptible to a number of diseases such as arthritis, heart disease, cancer, high blood pressure (called "hypertension"), diabetes, and cataracts. Older people also become more prone to infections such as bladder infections (called "urinary tract infections") and pneumonia. The person with Alzheimer's disease may develop one or more of these medical conditions. If the person requires medication, several issues arise such as remembering to take medication as prescribed, monitoring the condition being treated, staying alert to potential adverse side effects of the medications, and deciding when not to use medications to treat conditions that may develop in the terminal stages of the dementia.

Remembering to Take Medication as Prescribed

It is helpful to keep a medication log for the person with Alzheimer's disease. Write down the medications the person is taking, the doses and schedule, the expected outcome, potential side effects, and the length of time the person is expected to be taking each medication. Every medication has a brand name given by the company that makes and sells it and a generic name that is assigned to the compound regardless of the company that makes it. Write down both. Some doctors may only be familiar with the generic name, so it will make it easier to talk with the physician if you know the generic names of the medications being taken. Ask your pharmacist for help in filling out this log book.

Early in the course of the disease, something as simple as a tear-off calendar or a plastic pill box with compartments for each dose ("Med-Minders") may allow persons with Alzheimer's disease to continue to participate in managing their own medications. However, since memory problems are prominent in Alzheimer's disease, the person with dementia will almost always require some assistance with medications and eventually need someone to be responsible for making sure they are taken as the doctor has instructed.

Unless someone else is managing medications, memory problems can result in skipped or repeated doses of medication that can have serious consequences. For example, if the person with Alzheimer's disease also has diabetes and forgets to take a pill or inject insulin, dangerously elevated blood sugar levels may result, which can lead to many other problems including confusion, dehydration, and urinary incontinence. If, on the other hand, the person takes too many diabetes pills or too much insulin, the blood sugar can fall dangerously low and can cause confusion, agitation, seizures, and even death.

When giving a medication to your family member, give simple instructions and adequate liquid to aid swallowing. Check to see that the pill was swallowed and has not lodged in the cheek or under the tongue. Praise the person for a job well done. If the person is resistant to taking the medication, try to avoid an argument. Reasoning will probably not work, but if you wait a short while and try again, you may be successful. The person may forget the earlier refusal.

If your family member is unable to take pills, ask the physician if a liquid or other form is available. The nurse or pharmacist may also be able to give you suggestions about giving your family member medications.

Monitoring the Condition Being Treated

Some conditions, like diabetes, require close monitoring, especially if the person is taking insulin. This type of monitoring is usually too complex for the person with dementia to manage without assistance. Procuring services to assist in monitoring diabetes may be available through a home health agency (see Chapter 16) or you can be taught to do it.

Sometimes the need for medications changes. For example, persons with Alzheimer's disease often lose weight. Weight loss usually causes blood pressure to fall. When this happens, blood pressure medication needs to be lowered or discontinued. If it is not, a person's blood pressure may fall too low. This can cause confusion, dizziness (especially when standing), fatigue, and falls. If a person loses weight, their requirement for insulin or diabetes pills will also decrease.

When a medication is changed, record this and the reason in the medication log you are keeping.

Adverse Reactions to Medications

In addition to beneficial effects, all medications have the potential to cause undesired side effects. These are usually referred to as "adverse drug reactions" or "ADRs." ADRs may be difficult to detect in persons with Alz-heimer's disease because they cannot describe their problems.

Clues to the presence of an ADR include:

- Acute change in behavior.

- Increase in confusion.

- Urinary incontinence.

- Falling.

Call the doctor immediately if any of these symptoms occurs after beginning or changing the dose of a medication. If it is determined that the person did have an ADR, make note of this in your medication log so that you will know to avoid this medication in the future. This information is especially important if you see a physician who is not familiar with your family member, such as in an emergency room.

Since any medication can cause an ADR, it is best to have the person with Alzheimer's disease on the fewest number of medications possible. Be sure to review with the doctor at each visit which drugs are necessary and which ones might be eliminated. Also, the maintenance dose of almost all drugs is lower in older persons than in younger persons. Many medications can be used effectively at one-third to one-half the recommended dose for a younger person. Ask your doctor about reducing the dose of medications.

Medications Used to Treat a Condition Related to the Dementia

The person with Alzheimer's disease may develop a number of behavioral problems that are described in Chapter 11. Because of the potential of any medication to cause an ADR, whenever possible it is best to try to manage behavior problems without medication. For example, sometimes agitated behavior may be triggered by caffeine, alcohol, or physical discomfort. Try to determine the events that immediately preceded the behavior problem. It may be that this problem behavior can be avoided simply by eliminating coffee or alcohol or reminding your family member to empty their bladder every 2 or 3 hours to avoid the discomfort of a full bladder.

Sometimes, however, medications will help in managing certain behaviors that are caused by the dementia. The dose of any medication should be low at first, and the person receiving the medication should be observed closely. In particular, it will be important to monitor whether the specific condition the drug is being used for is affected by the medication. For example, if a medication is prescribed to help with anxiety, it might be helpful to write down how the person was behaving in the week before the medication was begun and again after taking the medication for a week. This information will guide the doctor and prevent the continued use of medications that are not helping. Some of the medications that may be prescribed are mentioned below. The generic name is first and the brand name is given in parentheses.

Medications for Anxiety

Medications taken to relieve anxiety are also called minor tranquilizers, anxiolytics, or nerve pills.

The types of medications prescribed for anxiety are benzodiazepines such as diazepam (Valium®) or lorazepam (Ativan®) and buspirone (Buspar®).

Side effects of such medications are confusion, drowsiness, worsening agitation, unsteadiness, and falling.

Medications for Depression

Medications taken to relieve depression are also called antidepressants.

The types of medications prescribed for depression are tricyclic antidepressants such as nortriptyline (Pamelor®), doxepin (Sinequan®), or desipramine (Norpramin®); and nontricyclic antidepressants such as trazedone (Desyrel®), fluoxetine (Prozac®), or sertraline (Zoloft®).

Side effects of some types of medications can cause drowsiness (e.g., doxepin, trazedone); and some types can cause agitation or anxiety (e.g., desipramine, fluoxetine).

There is general agreement among psychiatrists and geriatricians that the early antidepressants, amitriptyline (Elavil®) and imipramine (Tofranil®), should not be used to treat depression in older adults because they are more likely to cause adverse drug reactions than newer antidepressants but are no more effective.

Medications for Sleep

Medications taken to induce sleep are also called hypnotics or sleepers.

The types of medications prescribed for sleep are any of the benzodiazepines such as temazepam (Restoril®) or triazolam (Halcion®), chloral hydrate ("knock out pills"), antihistamines such as diphenhydramine (Benadryl®) or chlorpheniramine (Chlortrimeton®) and some antidepressants such as trazodone (Desyrel®) or doxepin (Sinequan®).

Side effects of such medications are confusion, drowsiness, worsening agitation, unsteadiness, falling, dry mouth, constipation, and difficulty urinating.

Medications for Hallucinations or Suspiciousness That Cause Extreme Fright

Medications taken for hallucinations or suspiciousness are also called major tranquilizers, antipsychotics, or neuroleptics.

The types of medications prescribed are haloperidol (Haldol®), thioridazine (Mellaril®), loxapine (Loxitane®), and molindone (Moban®).

Side effects of such medications are difficulty moving because of stiff muscles (called extrapyramidal side effects, which can look like Parkinson's disease), abnormal movements of the mouth, lips, and tongue (called tardive dyskinesia), restless movements of the legs (called akathisia), confusion, unsteadiness, a fall in blood pressure when standing, dry mouth, and difficulty urinating.

Other Medications Sometimes Used for Aggressive Behavior

One type of medications prescribed is beta-blockers such as propranolol (Inderal®).

Side effects of beta-blockers are low blood pressure, slow pulse, and depression.

Another type of medications is anticonvulsants such as carbamazepine (Tegretol®).

Side effects of anticonvulsants are dizziness, falling, and confusion.

Hospitalization

When persons with Alzheimer's disease are hospitalized for an acute illness (such as pneumonia) or for surgery (such as repair of a fractured hip), they frequently become extremely confused or agitated. This is caused by a number of factors including the illness or injury, strange environment, and hospital procedures. If they are restrained to prevent falls or to keep them from pulling out an IV line, they may become even more agitated. Families can help by sharing information about care with hospital staff, bringing in familiar items, and having frequent contact.

It is important that hospital staff know who is legally responsible for making medical decisions if your relative is no longer able to do so. If there is a personal guardian or a power of attorney for health care, be sure to leave that person's name and telephone number on the medical chart. You should also inform the staff if there are any medical interventions (such as a feeding tube or resuscitation) that are not authorized.

When people with Alzheimer's disease are bedridden for even a short period of time, walking may become difficult. Ask the staff to encourage walking as soon as it is safe. Request a physical therapy evaluation if there are problems.

It is not uncommon for patients to be discharged from hospitals before they have totally recovered from their illness or injury. Families need to be alert to this possibility and ask to see a social worker or discharge planner early to begin making plans. Here are some issues to discuss well before the discharge occurs:

- What community services are suggested when the person returns home? Who will make the referrals?

- What equipment, such as a walker or raised toilet seat, would be helpful and who will request it?

- If the person cannot return to the former living situation, what level of care is recommended (such as a nursing home or residential facility) and who will make the arrangements?

- If any special care is needed, such as changing a dressing on a wound, make sure you have clear written instructions.

- Ask what medications will be continued after discharge. Make sure you have a list of the names, doses, and times and that you have the prescriptions you need. If there are any new medications, ask for information about side effects.

Summary

Families caring for someone with a dementing illness need to become familiar with the health care system and serve as advocates to ensure adequate medical care is provided. They also need to become informed about community services that help maintain persons with Alzheimer's disease in the community. Providing care at home is the focus of the next chapter.

Chapter 16

Providing Care at Home

This chapter focuses on caring for someone with Alzheimer's disease at home. It includes evaluating what care is required, the importance of the family in providing care, and the types of assistance available through community agencies. It also describes how to find and initiate a new service and how to investigate funding sources.

The goal of most families is to keep the person with Alzheimer's disease at home as long as possible, but caring for someone with a dementing illness can exhaust even the most dedicated family. First of all, Alzheimer's disease usually lasts many years. Second, the disease requires a gradual change in family responsibilities from supervision, to assistance, to total care. The care itself is both physically and emotionally exhausting. For these reasons, caring for your relative is not something you can do alone. You need to enlist your entire family, doctor, supportive friends, neighbors, and community services.

Determining What Assistance You Need

Evaluating what help the person with Alzheimer's disease needs is complicated and depends both on the stage of the illness and the ability and willingness of family members to provide care.

Request a Group Meeting

At the time the illness is diagnosed, you should ask for a meeting with the doctor and any other staff who were involved in the evaluation. Questions to ask at that meeting are listed in Chapter 4.

Hire a Case Manager

Another way to arrange for an evaluation of the need for services is to hire a private "case manager" who is usually a social worker or a nurse. The case manager's responsibility is to visit your family member, evaluate everyday functioning, and suggest which services might be appropriate. If you wish, the case manager can also arrange and monitor these services, which might be especially helpful if you live a great distance from the person with Alzheimer's disease. The local Alzheimer's Association can help you locate a case manager. Because there are no certification or licensing standards for case managers in most states, it is wise to check references carefully.

Do Your Own Evaluation

The first step in doing your own evaluation is to examine the needs of the person with Alzheimer's disease. Decide whether your relative is completely independent, requires supervision, or requires total assistance with both personal care activities (dressing, bathing, toileting, grooming, eating, walking, and taking medications) and household tasks (laundry, cooking, cleaning, managing finances, shopping, and using the telephone). Look at safety issues such as smoking, driving, and falling.

Your answers will help determine what assistance is needed, how frequently, and whether you can safely leave your relative alone.

The second step is to evaluate the availability and capability of the family, especially the person who is responsible for most of the care (the "primary caregiver"). The plan of care will combine the needs of the person with dementia and the ability of family caregivers to meet those needs.

Plan Ahead

Because Alzheimer's disease is a progressive illness, it is important to try to anticipate what assistance may be required in the next phase of the illness. You should take time to collect information, apply for financial help, and put your relative's name on any waiting lists. If you wait until a crisis occurs, you may have fewer options, and you may be forced to make difficult decisions in a very short time.

Types of Assistance

Two main sources of help are available for the care of someone with a dementia: families and community services.

Families

Families provide most of the care of persons with Alzheimer's disease, often at the expense of their own health and other responsibilities. A spouse who is a primary caregiver is often reluctant to ask other family members for help for fear of being a "burden." Often other people in the family as well as friends and neighbors want to help but do not know what is needed and may be afraid to intrude.

Accepting help from others is an important and useful way to pace yourself so that you do not become exhausted or ill. You will also provide better care if you are rested and have regular time off from your responsibilities. Allowing other people to help also provides them with a concrete way of showing that they care about you and the person with Alzheimer's disease.

How Families Can Help

Your family or friends can either help you directly with the care of your relative or they can relieve you of some other responsibilities. Here are some suggestions for enlisting the assistance of others in providing care:

- Visiting with your family member.

- Going on a walk or to a special event.

- Helping with personal care such as bathing.

- Assisting with chores such as errands.

- Providing transportation.

- Bringing in meals on a regular basis.

- Helping with insurance forms or taxes.

- Paying for services such as day care.

- Arranging for periodic time away.

Emotional Support Is Important

Research has shown that emotional support from family and friends helps prevent burn-out by caregivers. Caring for someone with a progressive dementing illness can become lonely. Often constant supervision is required, and it becomes increasingly difficult to take someone with Alzheimer's disease along for a social outing or an errand. Because it is easy for the caregiver to become more and more isolated, phone calls, visits, letters, or flowers all are ways to stay in touch and show concern.

Community Services Are Helpful

As the disease progresses, most caregivers need to enlist the help of community agencies as well as family and friends to keep their relatives at home. Some families are reluctant to use formal community services. Locating and arranging services can be difficult, and some people are uncomfortable with having "strangers" in their homes. Others fear that they may lose control, worry about the expense, or feel ashamed about accepting welfare. Some people even think they have failed in their responsibilities if they ask for help. Use of community services, however, does not end the caregiver's involvement but instead re-quires the caregiver to act as the coordinator and advo-cate for the person needing care.

Many different kinds of community services have been developed to supplement the care provided by families and to allow them to have a much-needed break. The availability to services varies from state to state and between rural and urban areas. Because services are not organized in any logical way, families often become confused when they venture into the arena of formal services. Suggestions for locating services are provided later in this chapter. Once you do find a service that meets your needs, you will develop a network of people to call for advice.

Services Brought to Your Home

The following services can be provided directly in your home.

Telephone reassurance offers a daily call at an arranged time by a volunteer who provides social contact and checks on safety.

Friendly visitors are usually volunteers who drop in on a regular schedule to chat.

Library services include home delivery, large-print books, and "talking books." The latter is a free service from the Library of Congress. Contact your local library.

Personal emergency response systems are electronic devices worn by frail or confused older persons that enable them to call for help if they fall and are unable to reach the telephone. These may be helpful in early Alzheimer's disease but in the later stages of the illness the person may forget to wear the alarm or may not remember what it is for. Be sure to compare prices and beware of high pressure sales tactics.

Home modification programs install safety aides such as grab bars in the bathroom or railings on stairways to prevent falls.

Chore services provide help with heavy cleaning, repairs, or outdoor tasks.

Homemakers come to help with housekeeping tasks such as cleaning, laundry, meal preparation, or shopping.

Home health aides provide assistance with personal care such as bathing. They are trained and usually work under the supervision of a registered nurse in a home health agency.

Companions offer supervision and social contact. If the person with Alzheimer's disease requires help with personal care such as dressing or toileting, a companion is not appropriate.

Home-delivered meals or "meals on wheels" are useful if cooking is no longer a safe activity or if the person forgets to eat. This service provides at least one hot nutritious meal daily (usually 5 days a week).

Transportation services include door-to-door scheduled rides to destinations such as a doctor's office or an adult day care center.

Homesharing programs match persons who live alone but who need help or supervision with another person such as a college student who needs housing.

Professional services are provided by licensed home health agencies and require a doctor's order. They include care by registered nurses, physical or occupational therapists, speech pathologists, nutritionists, and social workers. Because persons with Alzheimer's disease usually do not need the skilled care provided by professionals, these services are of limited usefulness. Usually, only brief visits for a specified period of time are covered by Medicare. Private payment is always possible for those who can afford it.

Hospices offer care for terminally ill persons and their families, often in the home. Their goal is to keep patients comfortable. Some hospices are Medicare certified.

Services in Central Locations

The following programs require that you take your family member to the service.

Group nutrition sites are available in most communities and offer a hot meal and socialization. For someone in the early stages of Alzheimer's disease, a group meal is a way to keep in touch with others and have one balanced meal a day.

Senior centers provide interesting programs and activities for older persons. Like the group nutrition site, participants need to be independent.

Adult day care is a program of individualized services and activities in a group setting for adults who require supervision or assistance. Services include recreation, health monitoring, medication management, meals, assistance with personal care, therapy, transportation, and family support. Some adult day centers serve only persons with dementia.

Support groups for caregivers are an important source of information and encouragement from other people coping with similar situations. Contact the nearest Alzheimer's Association chapter for information.

Other Special Services

The following services may also be helpful.

Information and referral services link people to appropriate community programs. They are often provided by the local office on aging, the Area Agency on Aging, or United Way.

Protective services provide assistance in situations of suspected abuse or neglect. Often mandated by state law, they are usually the responsibility of a local government agency such as the office on aging or the social service department.

Mental health services provide assessment, treatment, and counseling for persons with dementia and their caregivers. They include community mental health centers as well as private practice mental health professionals such as psychiatrists, psychologists, psychiatric nurses, and social workers.

Respite services refer to care in or out of the home that allows caregivers to have time off from their responsibilities. Paid helpers, adult day care, or temporary placement in a residential facility or a nursing home are all forms of respite care.

Home Care and Adult Day Care Compared

The following are advantages of having services provided in your home:

- Your relative may function better in a familiar environment.

- The resistance, agitation, or anxiety that some persons with Alzheimer's disease have when getting ready for day care will be avoided.

Day care is an appropriate service when the person with dementia needs social stimulation, structured activities, or requires supervision while the caregiver is at work or has some time off. It has the following advantages:

- Day care almost always costs less per hour than home care.

- You will have your house to yourself. You can invite friends over, take a nap, or get some chores done without interruptions from either your relative or the home care worker.

- Day care offers more opportunity for socializing.

How to Begin a New Service

When you decide to use a community service, the following suggestions will help you get started:

- Collect information about all the available services.

- Make arrangements to use the service that best meets your needs.

- Provide information about the needs of your family member to the staff.

- Be prepared to deal with resistance to any new service.

- Decide on a trial period.

- Accept your responsibility for supervising and coordinating services.

Collecting Information

Obtaining information on the services in your community is an essential first step but may be a difficult, time-consuming, and frustrating task. Keep a log of the name and phone number of the agency or person you call, the date of contact, and the information received. Contact them again if you have further questions or if you do not receive the answers or materials you were promised.

Here are some general questions to ask about services when you call for information:

- What type of assistance is provided? How often is it provided? What geographic area is included?

- What eligibility criteria are there? For example, does the client have to be a certain age, have a particular medical diagnosis, or a specific income to be served?

- What is the application process? Is there an application form? Is an interview needed? Will an agency representative come to the home?

- What other suggestions of agencies or persons to contact do they have?

The following are good places to start your search for information about services:

State Office on Aging. Each state has an Office on Aging located in the state capitol.

Ombudsman. All states are required to have an Ombudsman responsible for monitoring quality of care in nursing homes. Some Ombudsman programs also include care in residential facilities and care provided in the home by home health agencies.

Area Agencies on Aging. States are subdivided into Area Agencies on Aging that coordinate programs and provide information to the public about community services in their regions.

National Eldercare Locator line. Sponsored by the National Association of Area Agencies on Aging, staff at this number provide information and referral to services in all states. Call 1-800-677-1116.

County or City Offices on Aging. Some county or city governments also have offices that serve the elderly (known as offices, councils, or commissions on aging; elderly services or affairs; senior citizen services). Look in the government listings in the telephone book.

Other Government Agencies. Services are often available from city or county health and social service or human service departments, which are listed under government in the telephone directory.

The Alzheimer's Association. Look for a listing of the local chapter in the telephone book or call 1-800-272-3900. The Alzheimer's Association has many free or low-cost publications on a variety of topics such as selecting home care or nursing homes.

Other sources of information. Try your doctor or nurse, hospital social workers or discharge planners, or the nearest senior center.

The telephone directory. In the beginning of the telephone book there may be a "self-help guide," information pages, or a local information and referral number. In the Yellow Pages, look for the following headings: home health, nurses, senior citizens, social service or human service organizations, and community or elderly services.

Making Arrangements for Services in Your Home

If you want to hire someone to care for your relative at home, you can either hire privately or use an agency.

How to Hire Private Help

Private help is usually less expensive than using an agency but it is often more time-consuming for families to find and supervise employees. Finding someone to hire privately can be done by word of mouth or by advertising. Sometimes local offices on aging or senior centers have lists of available persons. If you advertise, include the number of hours per day or week, the duties, your telephone number, and times you can be reached.

You will need to screen applicants on the telephone and then arrange for interviews. Find out:

- Where they have worked before.

- Whether they have experience caring for someone with Alzheimer's disease.

- Whether they are physically capable of the care required.

- Whether they have the skills to do what is expected; for example, do they know how to give a bath?

- Whether they are able to handle difficult behaviors or a crisis.

- Whether they will make a commitment to stay a certain length of time on this job.

Be sure to check the references of any applicant you are seriously considering. You will also need to develop a written contract that includes: hours and days of work, specific duties, pay per hour, fringe benefits, nonacceptable behavior, and termination.

How to Use an Agency

If you decide to use an agency instead of hiring private help, find out about its reputation by calling agencies or persons such as those listed previously in the section Collecting Information. Ask the following questions about the agency before starting any service:

- Is the agency licensed and/or certified?

- Are staff trained, supervised, and bonded?

- Have they cared for persons with dementia?

- Who is to be called about any concerns?

- Will they develop a written plan of care?

- How much will the service cost?

- Will they handle any insurance claims?

- Will they guarantee substitute staff?

- Will they assign one regular staff person?

- Do they have references available to you?

How to Choose an Adult Day Center

Make arrangements to visit the center. Ask these questions and take notes:

- Is it conveniently located and accessible?

- Do the hours of service fit your schedule?

- What is the ratio of staff to participants?

- What training or supervision of staff is provided?

- What professional staff is available?

- Who is to be called with questions or concerns?

- Can the staff dispense medications?

- Can the center handle incontinence?

- What is the cost per day?

- Are there any extra charges?

- Is there any available financial assistance?

- What activities or special events are planned?

- Is there special help such as bathing?

- What do they serve for lunch or snacks?

- How is transportation arranged?

- Does transportation cost extra?

- What happens in a medical emergency?

- Is there a written contract?

Describe the specific needs of your relative and ask how the day center would plan to meet those needs. Observe the other participants. Would your relative fit in? Do the other participants look involved or bored? Is the staff warm and friendly and interacting with participants? Is the center clean and comfortable? Do other participants have Alzheimer's disease?

Preparing Your Relative

Involving someone with Alzheimer's disease in the decision to use services depends on the stage of the illness and the amount of insight the person has. Be positive and reassuring. Keep explanations short. For example, say that it will be good to see some different people or that your doctor suggests it. Describe what is going to happen in clear simple terms. Reassure your family member that you will return.

Preparing the Staff

Whether you choose services in the home or in an adult day center you will need to help the staff understand your relative by answering the following questions:

- What responses are normal?

- What assistance is needed?

- What independent activities are possible?

- Which ways of providing help work best?

- What is the normal daily routine?

- What works best if your relative becomes upset?

- Which communication techniques are helpful?

- What should be done in an emergency?

Dealing with Resistance

Despite extensive preparation, many persons with dementia resist any change. They may initially object to having a home health aide give them baths or having to go to adult day centers. Remember that this is a normal reaction for someone with Alzheimer's disease who, given enough time, usually will adapt. Their adaptation will be easier if the services are more frequent. For example, if day care is scheduled only once a week, each time they return it may be a bewildering experience; if they go two or three times a week, it will more quickly become familiar and therefore less frightening.

Establishing a Trial Period

Decide to try this new service for at least 4 to 6 weeks before concluding whether it is beneficial to you or to your relative. Enlist the help of staff members in supporting you through this difficult trial period. During this time keep checking with the staff to see how the person is responding. It is not unusual for someone with Alzheimer's disease to be agitated or angry in your presence but to cooperate and enjoy the staff and activities when you are not there.

Supervising and Coordinating Services

Families have the important job of monitoring services once they begin. This can become quite complicated when more than one agency is involved. One way to make sure that everyone is working together and communicating well is to schedule periodic meetings of all the staff involved, to review how things are going, modify the plan if needed, and clarify everyone's role and responsibility. Do not be afraid to make suggestions. After all, you know your relative better than anyone else. On the other hand, professional staff who have experience in this area and who are not emotionally involved sometimes have a different perspective that may be very helpful.

Because a person with Alzheimer's disease is vulnerable and, in the later stages of the disease, unable to accurately describe any inappropriate care or report any abuse, continued family involvement in monitoring services is essential. This is especially difficult for families who live at a distance. Enlisting the help of trusted people such as neighbors, friends, or clergy to check periodically or employing a private case manager are possible solutions to this problem.

Paying For Services

The care of someone with Alzheimer's disease becomes more expensive as the disease progresses. For this reason the development of a long-range financial plan at the time of diagnosis is important (refer to Chapter 14).

You need to have a complete understanding of the costs and any possible funding sources before you initiate any service. It is not an easy task to sort through this maze. Keeping a log of the contacts you make and the information you receive will help you keep things straight.

The few public or private funding sources available to help pay the costs of caring for someone with Alzheimer's disease are listed in Chapter 14.

The cost of services is often a barrier to getting needed help. Some families do have sufficient resources but are so worried about the need for even more expensive care in the future that they refuse to spend any money on services they need in the present. This is "penny wise and pound foolish" because it may hasten the day when the caregiver is so exhausted that expensive nursing home care is the only option.

Summary

The main point of this chapter is that no one person can care for someone with Alzheimer's disease. There are many services available to assist families in keeping persons with dementia in their homes as long as possible. However, when more supervision and care are required, residential facilities should be explored. They are described in the next chapter.

Chapter 17

Residential Facilities

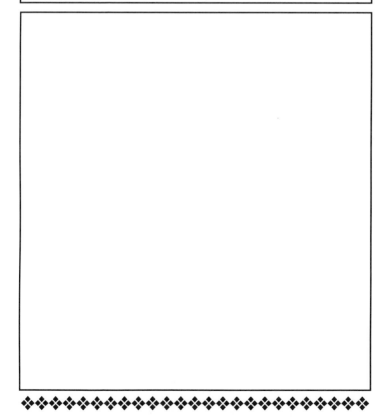

This chapter describes residential facilities that can be used as an intermediate step between home care and nursing home care. Indications for relocation, qualifications for a residential facility, and methods of payment are set forth as well as suggestions for helping the person with dementia adjust to new surroundings.

What are Residential Facilities

Residential facilities vary greatly from state to state in terms of size, cost, quality of care, staffing, services, and ownership. What residential facilities have in common is the provision of supervised group living to frail or disabled adults. All of them offer room and board; supervision; and some assistance with medications, dressing, or bathing.

Residential facilities are known by many different names:

- Adult foster care.
- Board and care.
- Group homes.
- Assisted living.
- Homes for adults.
- Adult family homes.
- Adult care facilities.
- Adult congregate living facilities.
- Domiciliary care homes.

Some are private homes in which residents are cared for by a family whereas others are large and have some professional staff. Those that serve only people with Alzheimer's disease usually have a higher ratio of staff to residents. Others serve both those with physical disabilities and dementing illnesses. Some will not accept any residents with the diagnosis of dementia. Others accept persons with dementia but refuse to accept particular difficult behavior such as wandering, incontinence, or angry outbursts.

The sponsorship of residential facilities varies greatly and includes: family operations, religious organizations, non-profit community agencies, large for-profit corporations, and nursing homes.

How Residential Facilities Differ From Nursing Homes

Residential facilities do not provide the constant medical supervision offered in nursing homes. Although nurses are sometimes available at scheduled times or "on call," there is no 24-hour nursing care.

How Residential Facilities Differ From Senior Apartments

Neither senior citizen apartments nor rooming houses provide the supervision and personal care that residential facilities offer. Persons with Alzheimer's disease who are having difficulty living alone in the community would probably not do well in a rooming house or a senior apartment.

Continuing Care or Life Care Communities

Continuing care or life care communities offer a full range of services including independent apartment living, assisted living, and long-term nursing home care. Residents are usually expected to be independent on admission, which sometimes excludes persons with a progressive illness such as Alzheimer's disease. There is usually a substantial entrance fee as well as a monthly fee and charges for extra services. If you are considering a continuing care community, make sure it accepts residents with Alzheimer's disease and has appropriate services at each level of care. Be sure to have a lawyer read over the contract. Ask whether care will continue to be provided if personal savings are exhausted. Check references.

Licensing

Most residential facilities are licensed by the state. However, in some states licensing requirements may be limited to fire safety or food preparation. Other states may have broader regulations concerning the number of staff and their training or types of services and activities. It is important that families visit and check references before making any decision. Good sources of information include the Alzheimer's Association, local social service department, office on aging, Area Agency on Aging or the state agency responsible for licensing and complaints.

When to Use a Residential Facility

There are many reasons for placement in a residential facility. Persons with Alzheimer's disease living alone often enter residential facilities sooner than those living with a caregiver. The need for 24-hour supervision, medication help, or companionship are common reasons.

For those who live with caregivers, exhaustion, illness, or death of the caregiver often prompts such a move. Other indications for placement in a residential facility include behavior problems or the inability to manage personal care.

Respite Care

Placement in a residential facility can also be short term as a respite for caregivers. Not all residential facilities offer respite care. Some require a minimum amount of time (such as 2 weeks). Usually advance notice is necessary, although some residential facilities accept respite placement in emergencies.

Plan Ahead

Because many of the best residential facilities are full and have waiting lists, it is wise to anticipate the need for a move. Even for those persons with Alzheimer's disease living with a caregiver, a back-up plan in the event of an emergency is recommended (see Chapter 9). Families should collect information about residential facilities, visit several, and get on the waiting list to increase the chance of an immediate admission in a crisis.

What to Look For in a Residential Facility

Call ahead to schedule visits to facilities that accept persons with Alzheimer's disease. Visit several facilities so you will have a basis for comparison. While you are there talk to residents as well as staff. Stay for a meal. Ask for names of families to call for references. Check to make sure the facility is licensed.

Share information about your relative. Discuss any special needs such as incontinence or behavior problems such as wandering to make sure the facility is equipped to provide needed care.

Inspect the Physical Facility

Go on a tour and observe whether the facility is clean and comfortable.

Bedrooms. Are there single or shared bedrooms? Are furnishings provided? Are personal possessions such as pictures or a favorite chair encouraged? Is there sufficient closet and storage space?

Bathrooms. Are bathrooms private or shared? Are they conveniently located, well labeled, clean, and free of odor? Are they equipped with grab bars or rails near the toilet and bathing areas? Do they have showers or tubs? How often are baths given?

Common Living Areas. Are the common areas large enough for visitors, television viewing, conversation, and resting? Are they clean and comfortable? Are there separate areas for smokers and nonsmokers?

Dining Room. Is it large enough for all the residents? Are mealtimes relaxed? Can residents sit where they like?

Kitchen. Is the kitchen clean? Is it available for the use of residents or visitors?

Grounds. Are the grounds attractive and inviting? Is it fenced? Is it near a busy street?

Safety. Ask about fire safety (smoke alarms, fire extinguishers, evacuation plans). Are staff trained in first aid? How are medical emergencies handled? Are there alarms on the outside doors to prevent wandering? Is smoking allowed? If so, is it restricted to certain areas or under supervision? Are there railings on all stairs? Are halls and stairs well lit and free of clutter?

Staff. What is the ratio of staff to residents during the day? At night? Is there a staff person awake at night? (important for residents who wander or become confused). Are staff friendly? Do they know the residents by name? Do they talk to them? Do they treat residents as adults? Do they make an effort to get to know new residents? Ask the administrator if staff is trained and experienced in caring for persons with dementia. Who supervises the staff? Who is to be called in an emergency or with concerns about care?

Services and Activities. Is there a plan of care for each resident that is reviewed periodically? Are family members invited to attend meetings when the plan of care is discussed? Does the facility control and dispense medications? Is written permission of the doctor needed? Is help with bathing, dressing, toileting, and eating available? Is there a limit on the number of hours of personal care each day? What personal care cannot be provided? Is there a variety of planned activity? Who plans and offers the activities? Do they include outings outside the facility? Is transportation to medical appointments or religious services arranged or provided by the facility?

Menus and Food. Are menus posted? Are they varied and well balanced? Does the food appear appetizing? Are snacks available? What happens if a resident is ill and unable to come to the dining room?

Residents. Are the residents clean and dressed? Do they converse with each other and with the staff? Do they seem comfortable in the common living areas or do they stay in their bedrooms? Do they participate in activities?

Cost and Admission Forms

There is great variation in cost from one residential facility to another. Some may cost less than living alone in an apartment whereas others may cost more than a nursing home.

Medicare does not pay for care in a residential facility. Some states have special programs to use Medicaid or SSI funds to pay for the care of people who have low incomes and assets. Some long-term care insurance plans pay for custodial care. In general, however, private payment is the usual funding source.

Be sure to explore costs carefully. Find out whether there is a basic monthly charge that covers everything or whether specific services (such as help with bathing) cost extra. Ask whether there is an entrance fee. Is it refundable if the move does not work out?

Read the written contract carefully before signing. Be sure you understand under what conditions and with what notice a resident can be asked to leave.

Usually there are required admission forms, some of which may need to be completed by the doctor. A chest X-ray or TB test may be necessary.

Adjustment to a Residential Facility

Change is difficult for someone with Alzheimer's disease who depends on familiar surroundings and people to provide cues. Resistance to a move is common and normal. Anxiety and confusion may increase temporarily but usually most people with Alzheimer's disease eventually adapt to their new surroundings.

Involving the person with dementia in the decision to move depends on the stage of the illness and the amount of insight the person has. Enlist the support of professionals, especially the doctor. Keep explanations simple. For example, say that you need help with care or that it is not safe to live alone. Unless it leads to increased anxiety, involve your relative in simple decisions about what to take. Familiar belongings such as photographs or mementos may help your relative feel at home and reduce confusion.

Prepare the Staff

You will need to help the staff understand the person with Alzheimer's disease. Explain what help is needed and what independent activity should be encouraged. Suggest approaches which work best if your relative becomes upset. Describe the normal daily routine and usual responses. Help staff with suggestions of ways to communicate.

Monitoring the Care

Although daily visits are not necessary, it is important to visit often enough to assure the care is adequate and to let your relative know you are still involved. Try to divide visiting responsibilities among family and friends so that visits are spread out. Visiting at different times will also enable you to get to know the staff on different shifts. If you live at a distance and cannot visit often, stay in touch by phone or ask others you trust to visit for you.

If visiting is painful because the person with dementia seems unhappy or begs to come home, talk to the staff. It is not unusual for a person with Alzheimer's disease to be agitated or unhappy in your presence but to enjoy the facility and staff when you are not there.

Developing good relationships with staff may ensure better care and make it easier to share any concerns you may have. It is difficult to let go and accept that the facility's care is not going to be the same as your care. Try to give positive feedback and restrict complaints to urgent matters as opposed to differences in style. If you have serious concerns, schedule a meeting with the person in charge.

Adjustment of Family

Making the decision to place someone in a residential facility is often a painful process. It helps if everyone shares in the decision making. It is common for families to feel a mixture of relief, guilt, loss, and loneliness after such a move. This is a time when the caregiver needs extra support from the rest of the family and friends.

Summary

Residential facilities offer care for persons with dementia who can no longer live in the community but who do not require 24-hour nursing home care. When continuous skilled nursing care is needed, nursing homes are usually the only option. Nursing homes are the topic of the next chapter.

Chapter 18

Nursing Homes

The focus of this chapter is nursing homes. It includes reasons for nursing home placement and ways to find and pay for nursing home care. Special Alzheimer's units, adjustment to the move, and working with staff are also discussed in this chapter.

When to Use a Nursing Home

Although not every person who has Alzheimer's disease requires nursing home care, placement is often the only option in the later stage of the illness as the need for physical care increases. Because it is impossible at the beginning of Alzheimer's disease to predict either the course of the illness or the continued availability of family caregivers, it is wise to avoid making a promise never to use a nursing home.

Most families are dedicated to providing care at home for as long as possible. Premature placement in nursing homes is rare. In fact, most families postpone placement because of a deep sense of obligation as well as concern about cost and quality of care. The community services described in Chapter 16 can often help delay the need for nursing home care. However, when the painful decision is made it is usually because all other options have been exhausted.

Often nursing home placement is precipitated by an event that is beyond the control of families. Common reasons for placement include:

- Need for 24-hour nursing and medical monitoring.

- Illness or death of the primary caregiver.

- Lack of sufficient or affordable community services.

- Exhausting heavy physical care.

- Safety issues such as wandering.

- Difficult behaviors such as combativeness.

- Need for respite care (short-term placement).

Because there are many situations such as those listed above, when a nursing home is the most appropriate setting placing someone should not be seen as failure but rather as the responsible choice to assure needed care.

Plan Ahead

It is wise to anticipate the need for possible nursing home placement ahead of time. The selection of a nursing home is complicated and time consuming. Many nursing homes have waiting lists. For this reason making a nursing home placement in a crisis often means having to accept whatever is available regardless of location and quality of care.

The importance of planning ahead is covered in Chapter 9. The need for financial and legal planning for long-term care is addressed in Chapter 14. It is helpful for families to identify ahead of time what level of care could not be managed at home. This commonly includes management of incontinence, wandering, aggressive behavior, and care of someone who is bedridden. Some families decide to use a nursing home when the person with Alzheimer's disease ceases to recognize either family or home.

There are times when the decision to use a nursing home is clear (such as the illness of the caregiver), and there are many situations where the decision is much harder to make. It is in these situations that families are most likely to disagree about whether to seek nursing home care. A family meeting to discuss the pros and cons of placement, assessing the needs of both the person with Alzheimer's disease and the primary caregiver, may be helpful. Ask your doctor or another professional's advice. Talk about your dilemma in a support group. Chances are there will be other families who have struggled with a very similar decision. Reaching a consensus in the family about placement is important to provide emotional support to the primary caregiver and to help alleviate later feelings of guilt about the decision.

Investigate Admission Requirements

Although the rules about nursing home admissions vary greatly between states and facilities, there are several general issues to be resolved before beginning to look. They include:

Is nursing home placement necessary? Some states have preadmission screening programs (usually run by the local social service department) to make sure people are not being inappropriately placed in nursing homes. Certain levels of care are often required for funding such as Medicaid to be approved. Your doctor, nurse, or social worker will be able to help determine whether nursing home care is needed.

How will the care be funded? If a public source of funding (such as Medicaid) is necessary, the care will need to meet the medical criteria. Families should keep in mind that it is often difficult to get into a nursing home on Medicaid without an initial period of private pay.

Are there legal problems with placement? If the person with dementia is too confused to participate in the decision or sign the admission papers, the nursing home may allow the family to sign the forms and arrange the placement. Some nursing homes, however, require a durable power of attorney for health care giving specific authority for nursing home admission as well as a durable power of attorney for finances to assure payment. If these documents are not available, guardianship and a specific court order for placement may be needed (refer to Chapter 14).

How to Choose a Nursing Home

Nursing homes vary greatly in quality of care, size, cost, ownership, types of services, and mix of residents. Sponsorship includes religious organizations, public agencies, nonprofit community groups and for-profit corporations. Some nursing homes are local individual operations whereas others are part of national chains. Some accept a wide range of disabilities including residents with dementing illnesses whereas others exclude persons with Alzheimer's disease. Some will only take private-paying residents whereas others admit persons on Medicare or Medicaid. All nursing homes are licensed by the state, and those that accept Medicare and Medicaid are also certified by those programs.

The first step in choosing a nursing home is to select several in the area that provide good quality care. Nursing homes are listed in the Yellow Pages telephone directory.

Good sources of information about quality are the Alzheimer's Association, your doctor, hospital social workers, clergy, and the local office on aging.

Call the admissions person for each nursing home on your list. Ask the following questions:

- Are residents with Alzheimer's disease admitted?

- Is Medicaid as a payment source accepted?

- Is there an opening or a waiting list?

Narrow your list based on the above information. If an immediate placement is not needed, the length of the waiting list may not be important. If the person has sufficient resources to pay privately for many years, whether the home takes Medicaid funding may not be an issue.

Before you visit, decide what aspects of care are most important. For example, the activity program may not be significant for a resident who is bedridden or too confused to participate. Think about the next stage of the illness and ask whether the facility will be able to meet future as well as current needs. Clarify what behavior or care the facility is not able to manage.

Schedule a Visit

It is important to visit several nursing homes for comparison. Take someone with you for support and help in the evaluation. Schedule at least an hour for each visit and stay for the noon meal if possible. Take a tour of the whole facility. Observe residents and staff as well as the physical plant. Meet with the director of nursing, the social worker, and the administrator. Honestly describe your relative's need for care. Take notes and collect any written information such as fee schedules.

The following section suggests ways to evaluate and compare nursing homes.

Licensure. Ask to see the facility's state license as well as Medicaid and Medicare certificates. The latest report by the state licensing agency is a public document that should be available to you. You can also call the state Ombudsman for information on the quality of care (see Chapter 16). Bear in mind that the reputations of nursing homes can change quickly for better or worse with a change in administration or ownership.

Location. Is the nursing home easily accessible for visits by family or friends? Are the outside grounds inviting? Are there places to sit and walk?

General Atmosphere. Is the facility clean, in good repair, and free of odor? Are there smoke-free areas? Is the staff friendly and cheerful? Do they know the residents by name? Are the furnishings attractive and comfortable? Are staff receptive to your questions?

Residents. Residents should be dressed, clean, well groomed, and treated with dignity by staff. Privacy should be respected. Assess whether residents seem sedated or whether they are alert.

Staff. Nursing homes have professional staff such as an administrator, medical director, registered nurses, social workers, attending physicians, therapists (physical, occupational, and speech), and dietitians. Find out what these staff do, how long they have been there, what training and experience they have working with people with Alzheimer's disease, how they work with families, and how responsive and interested they are in your relative's need for care.

The nonprofessional staff, such as nursing assistants, provide most of the direct care of residents. Ask about their training, supervision, and experience working with dementing illnesses. Find out about staff turnover at this level. Ask how many residents are assigned to each nursing assistant.

Medical Services. Ask whether there is a registered nurse on duty 24 hours a day and if there is a physician available in an emergency. Find out how often the medical director visits the facility, whether residents are allowed to keep their private doctors, and how often doctors are required to see each resident. Ask about which hospital is used in an emergency. Discuss the individual care plans for each resident and ask whether families are invited to staff meetings when their relatives' care plans are being reviewed.

Philosophy. Inquire about the facility's philosophy concerning the use of medications or restraints to manage difficult behaviors. Restraints must be ordered by the doctor and checked frequently. Investigate policies concerning residents who resist eating or drinking. Ask if a durable power of attorney for health care that specifically prohibits feeding tubes or other aggressive treatment will be honored.

Other Services. Observe what activities are occurring, whether there is an events calendar and whether residents are actually participating. Ask about religious services and visits by clergy. Find out about the provision of transportation to medical appointments. Is there a barber and beauty shop? Is personal laundry done by the facility? How should clothes be marked? Does the facility have a volunteer program that involves the local community?

Family. How is family participation encouraged? Are there regular family meetings with staff? Who on the staff helps families with concerns about care or other issues such as applying for Medicaid? Ask if families are consulted when a room or roommate change is made. Find out about visiting hours and the procedures for taking someone out of the facility for a brief visit or overnight.

Safety. Find out whether there are regular fire drills and an evacuation plan. Are there fire alarms, extinguishers, a sprinkler system, and clearly marked exits? Observe whether there are handrails along the halls and in the bathrooms. Is the lighting adequate and are the hallways free of clutter?

Meals. Is the dining room pleasant? Mealtime relaxed? Food attractively served? Are residents encouraged to eat in the central dining room? Review the posted menu and note the variety of foods. Ask whether special diets are available. What about snacks between meals? Is there help available for those who cannot feed themselves? What provisions are made for bedridden residents?

Bedrooms. Ask how many residents share a bedroom and if furnishings are provided. Are personal items encouraged? Find out whether there is adequate storage space. Look for a call button near the bed. Discuss roommate selection practices.

Bathrooms. Are bathrooms easily accessible, clean, and equipped with call buttons? Ask how many residents share each bathroom, how privacy is assured, and how often baths are given.

Common Rooms. Are there sufficient lounge and activity rooms? Are they inviting? Are residents using them or do they stay in their own rooms? Is there space for private family visiting?

Once you have visited several facilities you will be able to evaluate which nursing home is best able to provide needed care, how payment is to be made, and how soon placement is possible.

Admission Papers

The admission papers usually include a medical form to be completed by the doctor and financial and personal information to be completed by the family. A chest X-ray or a TB skin test is often required. It is also necessary to identify a doctor who will care for the person in the nursing home. Be sure that any advance directives (see Chapter 14) such as a durable power of attorney for health care are put in the medical record at the nurses station so staff will know what to do and who to call in an emergency.

Waiting Lists

If you are planning ahead for a future placement, discuss the waiting list policy. Often it requires filling out at least some of the admission papers and making a deposit that may or may not be refundable. Ask how many times you are allowed to turn down an admission before the name is removed from the waiting list.

Special Alzheimer's Units

Some nursing homes have units specifically for residents with Alzheimer's disease or other dementing illnesses. Carefully explore whether the unit is simply a place where the most difficult residents are put or if it really meets the special needs of residents with dementia. Special units do not necessarily provide better care and are not appropriate for all persons with a dementing illness.

Here are some questions to ask about a special unit:

• How many residents are in the special unit?

• Are there more staff per resident during all shifts?

• What is the staff turnover on this unit?

• Are all staff trained specifically in caring for persons with dementing illnesses?

• Is the unit designed to care for residents only at a specific stage of Alzheimer's disease? If so, what happens when the illness progresses? Who determines when a resident is moved? What are the criteria? Where do they go?

• Observe the atmosphere. Is it calm and peaceful? Is there a predictable daily schedule? Are activities tailored to persons with Alzheimer's disease? Do residents eat in their own dining room or in the central dining room with all the residents of the facility?

• What provisions have been made for wanderers (such as alarms or locks on the doors)? Is there an enclosed outside area?

• What is the philosophy on the use of medications and restraints for behavior management? Do you see many residents who appear sedated or are restrained?

• Does the special unit cost more per day? Is it worth the extra cost? Will Medicaid pay this cost?

Residents who may not belong in a special unit include those who have other illnesses (such as diabetes) that may be better managed in a medical unit and those who are so confused they can no longer benefit from special activities.

Payment

Because nursing homes are expensive, most families find the costs of long-term placement prohibitive. Other than Medicaid, there are few funding sources beyond private payment. Furthermore, funding often requires a certain level of care.

Levels of Care

There are three basic levels of care. Many nursing homes only offer skilled and intermediate care, not custodial care.

Skilled nursing care (often referred to as SNF for "skilled nursing facility") provides 24-hour a day care by a registered nurse. Examples of skilled nursing care include injections, dressing changes, and close observation of residents who are medically unstable.

Intermediate care provides some nursing care but not on a round-the-clock basis.

Custodial care provides supervision and help with personal care such as bathing or eating but little or no medical care.

Many persons with Alzheimer's disease are in good physical health and only require custodial care, which neither Medicaid nor most private insurance policies will cover. The only options for care in such situations are residential facilities (described in Chapter 17) or care at home (see Chapter 16).

Sources of Payment

The importance of financial planning, including sources of payment, is described in Chapter 14. None of the following funding sources are likely to pay for nursing home care (see the illustration on p. 272):

Medicare. This requires daily skilled care or rehabilitation as well as an initial hospitalization (which is often difficult to justify unless there is an acute illness in addition to the dementia). The nursing home must be Medicare certified. The number of covered days is limited. Custodial care is not covered.

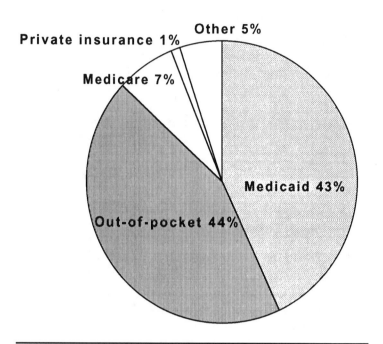

Nursing home costs. (Source: HCFA, 1989 data.)

Private Insurance. Some policies exclude dementia and do not pay for custodial care.

Veterans Administration (VA). Placement in a VA nursing home or payment by the VA for temporary care in a community nursing home is possible for certain veterans who meet eligibility criteria.

The most common sources of payment are private pay and Medicaid. Many persons pay privately until their assets are spent down to the allowed levels and then apply for Medicaid (refer to Chapter 14).

Medicaid. Also known as Medical Assistance or Title 19, Medicaid is a combined federal and state program that has strict financial and medical eligibility requirements. Eligibility and covered services vary from state to state. Usually the social service or welfare department determines eligibility. Not all nursing homes accept residents on Medicaid because payments are usually low. Residents on Medicaid are allowed to have a small personal allowance every month but otherwise their income is used to pay for the cost of care, and Medicaid supplements the difference.

States vary in terms of the income and assets the "community spouse" is allowed to keep when the spouse with Alzheimer's disease enters a nursing home on Medicaid. Medicaid does not require that the home be sold as long as the community spouse lives there. Part of the financial and legal planning recommended in Chapter 14 includes careful preparation for the financial survival of the community spouse when nursing home placement is needed.

Special questions to ask the nursing home admissions staff about Medicaid:

- Is the business office or other staff available to help with the Medicaid application?

- Will the nursing home keep residents on Medicaid once private funds are exhausted?

- Is a minimum period of private pay needed before Medicaid is accepted?

- Are residents on Medicaid moved to a special section of the home?

- Does the quality of care for residents on Medicaid differ from private pay residents?

Determining the Cost

An important part of your visit to each nursing home will be to ask questions about charges. Find out the basic daily rate and what it includes. Ask about additional charges such as incontinence supplies, laundry, phone, transportation, or equipment such as wheelchairs. Determine whether the cost will increase as the disease progresses.

If you are given a contract, ask a lawyer to review it. Clarify the following questions:

- If a relative is asked to co-sign the contract, does this obligate the family to pay for care if other funding sources (such as Medicare or private resources) are exhausted?

- What is the state law on financial responsibility of families?

- What happens if the resident is transferred to a hospital? Is there a "bed hold"? For how long? Who pays for the bed hold? How much does it cost?

- Clarify under what circumstances a resident may be asked to leave. How much notice is required? What is the nursing home's responsibility for helping the family locate another acceptable facility? What is the appeal process?

Be aware that it is illegal for nursing homes to ask for advance payment for residents on Medicare or Medicaid.

Moving to a Nursing Home

Any change is difficult for someone with Alzheimer's disease. Expect a longer period of adjustment with the possibility of increased agitation, confusion, anger, or withdrawal. Keep explanations simple ("you need the care of a nurse"). Provide staff with suggestions about care (see Chapters 16 and 17).

Bring familiar items such as family pictures or a favorite afghan to personalize the room. Because persons with Alzheimer's disease often can no longer present their own histories, help the staff get to know them as they once were. Display a photo of a trophy fish, favorite vacation spot, special award, or something they made to stimulate conversation with staff or visitors.

On the day of the move bring a relative or friend with you for support. Arrange with the staff in advance when to come and how long to stay. Keep in touch with the staff by phone after you leave and consult them about the timing of the first visit.

Families commonly experience conflicting emotions at the time of a nursing home placement. Feelings include guilt, relief, anger, loneliness, and anxiety. It is hard to give up control to strangers for the care of someone you love. Grief over the loss of the previous relationship and the responsibilities of being the caregiver are common. It takes time to adjust and to recuperate from the demands of caregiving. This is a time when caregivers especially need emotional support from family and friends. Support groups may also be helpful.

Visiting

Visiting may be difficult. The nursing home resident may seem unhappy and angry or beg to come home or accuse you of abandonment. If this happens be sure to check with the staff to see how your relative is when you are not there. People with Alzheimer's disease commonly forget visits the minute they are over and may claim that you have not visited for weeks. Some family or friends may find visiting too painful or depressing. Others may not know what to do when they visit. Going on a walk, listening to favorite music, reading a simple story or looking at family photos are all possibilities.

The frequency of visits depends on the health and other responsibilities of family and friends as well as the distance. Try to arrange a visiting schedule so not everyone comes at once. Caregivers who visit every day all day may need encouragement to take time for themselves and allow staff to provide care. If you have concerns about visiting, talk to the social worker or nurse.

Working with the Staff

Developing a good relationship with the staff is extreme-ly important. Visit at different times of day to get to know the staff on all three shifts. Keep in regular contact by phone if you live at a distance. Ask to participate in care plan meetings. Provide positive feedback.

If you have questions or concerns about the quality of care, talk with the nurse or social worker. Involve your doctor or the administrator if necessary. Ask for a special meeting if you feel it would be helpful. If the staff is not responsive to your concerns, contact the state Ombudsman who monitors care in nursing homes (see Chapter 16).

Summary

Placement in a nursing home is often a difficult decision for families, not only because of the expense but also because it often signals the terminal stage of the illness. Death is the inevitable last event in the long progression of Alzheimer's disease and is the subject of the next and final chapter of this book.

Chapter 19

Death

Alzheimer's disease is a terminal illness that eventually results in death. This chapter describes causes of death, decisions facing families regarding care in the terminal stage, and the experience of families when death occurs.

Although it is not possible to predict the rate of progression of Alzheimer's disease, the terminal stage of the illness has some general characteristics that are described in Chapter 5.

Cause of Death

Our sophisticated health care technology is capable of either helping people live longer or prolonging dying. This has resulted in many extremely complicated ethical and legal dilemmas as families and health care professionals struggle to determine how to measure quality of life, prevent harm and suffering, and determine what is in the best interest of the person who is ill.

Because of problems with nutrition, physical conditioning, and hygiene, persons with advanced Alzheimer's disease are less resistant to illness or injuries. Death for someone with Alzheimer's disease is usually caused by one of the following:

- Complications of late-stage Alzheimer's disease such as pneumonia, urinary tract infection, or skin breakdown (decubitus ulcers).

- Other acute or chronic illnesses such as heart disease, cancer, or diabetes.

Other Causes of Death

Occasionally persons with dementia die from causes such as car accidents, falls, or medication accidents. In the early stage of Alzheimer's disease some commit suicide (see Chapter 10). Sometimes suicide is a clear-minded decision to end life in anticipation of future decline. Often, however, suicide is caused by a clinical depression that might respond to treatment. At any sign of depression or suicide arrange for an immediate evaluation by a physician.

Helping someone commit suicide, known as assisted suicide, is almost always illegal even when the motive is humanitarian. It is an extremely controversial topic in our society and becomes particularly complicated in the case of someone with dementia. It is difficult to assess whether the person really prefers death, is responding to pressure from others, or has a treatable depression. Further information on this topic can be found in the library or from the Hemlock Society, PO Box 11830, Eugene OR 97440, telephone 1-800-247-7421.

Decisions about Death

Plan Ahead

It is widely recognized that competent persons have the right to refuse medical treatment. Because persons with late-stage Alzheimer's disease are usually unable to make their own decisions, the best way to assure that their wishes are followed is to discuss these issues early when they are still competent and have them prepare written advance medical directives including a durable power of attorney for health care or a living will to provide instructions (see Chapter 14). Written instructions help reduce the chance of conflict between family members or between family and health care providers and may also alleviate any guilt that relatives may feel later about their decisions.

Guardianship

Informal decisions by family about medical treatment are not always honored by hospitals, nursing homes, or doc tors. This is particularly true when there are no written instructions and/or when there is conflict among family members about what to do. In such situations it may be necessary to petition the court to appoint a guardian who will have the legal authority to make all medical decisions (see Chapter 14).

Issues in the Terminal Stage

Families need to openly discuss goals of medical treatment in the terminal stage. If the goal is to prolong life, different decisions may be called for than if it is to provide comfort. If you need more information or help in deciding on a course of action, ask for a meeting with your doctor. Your clergy may also be helpful. Many hospitals and nursing homes also have ethics committees that help resolve differences in such situations. Information on specific laws in each state can be obtained from Choice in Dying, Inc., 200 Varick Street, 10th floor, New York, NY 10014, telephone 212-366-5540. It also maintains a registry service for advance directives.

The following are possible issues that should be discussed well before a crisis occurs and included in the written advance medical directives:

- If the heart stops, should resuscitation (CPR) be attempted?

- If the kidneys fail, should dialysis be started?

- If pneumonia develops, should it be treated aggressively, which sometimes involves hospitalization, intravenous (IV) antibiotics, and restraints to keep the IV from being pulled out?

- If swallowing is a problem, should a feeding tube be put in?

- If breathing becomes difficult, should oxygen or a breathing machine (respirator) be used?

- If a hip is fractured, should surgery be performed?

- If falling is a risk, should restraints be used?

- If another illness such as cancer develops, should it be treated aggressively?

- Should preventive health care such as yearly flu shots be continued?

Death in an Institution

Many persons in the terminal stage are in nursing homes or hospitals. It is important to be sure that the durable power of attorney, living will, and any other written instructions be placed in the medical chart so staff on all shifts know what to do in a crisis.

Death at Home

If it appears that death will occur at home, families need to know beforehand what to do. Hospice programs that provide care for terminally ill persons usually have procedures to follow at the time of death. If there is no hospice care, ask your doctor, nurse, social worker, home care agency, coroner, or funeral home director whom to notify at the time of death. Keep in mind that if you dial an emergency number such as 911, the rescue squad may be required by law to attempt resuscitation even if there are written instructions to the contrary.

Identify the Cause of Death

If the death is caused directly or indirectly by Alzheimer's disease or another dementing illness, it is important that this be listed on the death certificate. This will identify the magnitude of the problem to public officials and help justify funds for research and health care in the future.

Autopsy

An autopsy of the brain at the time of death is the only way to confirm the diagnosis of Alzheimer's disease. The brain tissue is examined under a microscope to see if it exhibits the characteristic changes of the illness described in Chapter 5. Families receive a written report of the findings.

Families often agree to an autopsy for the following reasons:

- To be sure the diagnosis was correct.

- To have accurate family health records. If other relatives develop dementia, this information is important in the diagnosis.

- To assist in research relating to the cause and future treatment of Alzheimer's disease. Without brain tissue, research cannot move forward.

- To identify the correct cause of death on the death certificate.

The decision to have an autopsy should be discussed by the family ahead of time. Sometimes autopsies are free if they are part of a research grant or done at a university. Find out about costs of both the autopsy itself and transportation of the body. If you decide to have an autopsy, inform your doctor, hospital or nursing home, and funeral home of your intention. Contact the nearest Alzheimer's Association for information about its Autopsy Assistance Network and nearest autopsy site.

Grief

Grief is a normal response to loss. Unlike a sudden death, the grief experienced by relatives of persons with Alzheimer's disease often begins at the time of the diagnosis and continues throughout the illness. This is known as anticipatory grief and is a result of the many losses that come with dementia such as:

- Loss of future dreams, particularly for the spouse.

- Loss of the past, especially for children.

- Loss of companionship.

- Change in roles.

- Loss of financial security.

- Anticipation of further losses and eventual death.

For many families there are two deaths to grieve: the slow death of the unique personality followed by the physical death of the body. It is not uncommon for families to wish for death to come and then feel guilty about having such thoughts. Hoping for death is a normal reaction when a loved one is suffering.

Some family members, on the other hand, are unable to come to terms with the fact that Alzheimer's disease is a terminal illness until death actually occurs. Others find the slow death so painful to watch that they distance themselves from the process. There is no right way to handle this challenge. The reaction of each individual in the family depends on factors such as personality, past relationship with the person who is ill, communication patterns, and the length of the illness.

Common Grief Reactions

Although grief is an experience unique to each person, certain feelings are common. They include:

- Shock

- Disbelief

- Anger

- Guilt

- Depression

- Loneliness

Despite the fact that grief varies from person to person, it is usually most intense immediately after the death and for the next several months. Even after that, however, ups and downs are common during the first year although the intensity usually diminishes.

Grief Complications

For some people, grief continues at an intense level rather than abating with the passage of time. If prolonged acute grief begins to interfere with everyday functioning, a professional evaluation is indicated. The line between grief and depression is a fine one, and if depression develops it needs treatment (see Chapter 10).

Coping with Grief

Here are some suggestions for coping with grief:

- Express your feelings. Cry if you feel like it.

- Look for support from others.

- Take care of yourself. Rest, eat a well-balanced diet, get regular exercise, and see your doctor.

- Accept that grief is a normal response to loss.

For caregivers of persons with Alzheimer's disease, death brings both relief from the relentless demands of caregiving as well as the loss of responsibility that consumed many hours of each day. Many caregivers have given up friends, activities, and interests. It is not an easy matter to pick up life where you left off years earlier. It may take time, patience, and small tentative steps before it feels comfortable to enjoy life again.

Sources of Help

Many communities offer support groups for people coping with death of a loved one. These are often offered by churches, hospices, hospitals, counseling agencies, or funeral homes. There are also organizations such as widowed persons groups that offer support and activities. Contact the Alzheimer's Association, local office on aging, or your clergy for information.

Summary

The terminal stage brings with it many difficult decisions for families. It also brings grief as death is anticipated. Emotional support is important before and after death as caregivers adjust to their loss.

Index

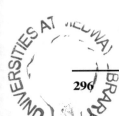